"There is a lot we can do with our mental efforts to alter the machinery of the brain. We now know that cognitive training empowers us to alter the hunger mechanism of the brain so that we can effectively prevent ourselves from habitual and mindless overeating."

—Jeffrey M. Schwartz, MD, Research Professor of Psychiatry, UCLA School of Medicine, Author of *Brain Lock, The Mind and the Brain*

D1166369

THINK
yourself THIN

The REVOLUTIONARY SELF-HYPNOSIS
SECRET to PERMANENT WEIGHT LOSS

Darcy D. Buehler, Ph.D.

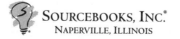
SOURCEBOOKS, INC.®
NAPERVILLE, ILLINOIS

Copyright © 2007 by Darcy Buehler
Cover and internal design © 2007 by Sourcebooks, Inc.
Cover photo © Corbis
Internal photos © Corbis and Artville

Sourcebooks and the colophon are registered trademarks of Sourcebooks, Inc.
All rights reserved. No part of this book may be reproduced in any form or by any elec-
tronic or mechanical means including information storage and retrieval systems—except in
the case of brief quotations embodied in critical articles or reviews—without permission in
writing from its publisher, Sourcebooks, Inc.

All brand names and product names used in this book are trademarks, registered trademarks,
or trade names of their respective holders. Sourcebooks, Inc. is not associated with any product or vendor in this book.

This book is not intended as a substitute for medical advice from a qualified physician. The
intent of this book is to provide accurate general information in regard to the subject matter covered. If medical advice or other expert help is needed, the services of an appropriate
medical professional should be sought.

Published by Sourcebooks, Inc.
P.O. Box 4410, Naperville, Illinois 60567-4410
(630) 961-3900
FAX: (630) 961-2168
www.sourcebooks.com

Originally published in 2004 as *Think Yourself Thin*, ISBN 1-879915-14-6

Library of Congress Cataloging-in-Publication Data
Buehler, Darcy D.
    Think Yourself Thin with CD: the Revolutionary Self-hypnosis Secret to Permanent
Weight Loss / Darcy D. Buehler.
        p. cm.
    Rev. ed. of: Think Yourself Thin, 2004.
    Includes bibliographical references.
    ISBN-13: 978-1-4022-0799-0
    ISBN-10: 1-4022-0799-9
    1. Weight loss. 2. Autogenic training. 3. Mind and body. I. Buehler, Darcy D. Think
yourself thin. II. Title.

RM222.2.B83 2007
613.2'5—dc22

                                                          2006027809

Printed and bound in the United States of America
VP 10 9 8 7 6 5 4 3 2 1

Author's Note

The information in this book is given to help you make informed decisions about how to achieve permanent weight loss. As with any weight loss program, you should consult your physician regarding any changes you choose to make as a result of following procedures or suggestions offered in this program. The author and publisher disclaim any liability, personal or otherwise, as a result of this program.

CENTRAL ARKANSAS LIBRARY SYSTEM
ADOLPHINE FLETCHER TERRY BRANCH
LITTLE ROCK, ARKANSAS

To my daughter, Kallie Hapgood—every mother's dream

Acknowledgments

First and foremost, I want to thank my editor, Deb Werksman, for believing in a first-time author with a new idea.

I want to thank my dear friend, Carol Russell, who was the first person to read the manuscript and gave me the encouragement to move forward with this project. Since that time, the support and suggestions from my parents, Bruce and Jacque Buehler, and my daughter, Kallie Hapgood, have been invaluable. In addition to the aforementioned, the following friends played a major role in helping me bring this book to you: Jane Luellen, Jay Allbaugh, Kevin Brown, Reuben Saunders, Bonnie Bing, Kim Herres, Jamie Coulter, Greg Buell, Susan Herbel, Terry O'Toole, Janet Neitzel, Gary Krause, Fun O'Neal, Karen Rogers, Jon and Myrna Roe, Fay Yates, and Andrea Taylor.

To all of them I express my love and gratitude.

Audio CD Contents

Track 1. Chapter 1 Self-hypnosis Script:
Rewiring Your Brain

Track 2. Chapter 2 Self-hypnosis Script:
This Precious Moment

Track 3. Chapter 3 Self-hypnosis Script:
Decision Making

Track 4. Chapter 4 Self-hypnosis Script:
Die Young as Late in Life as Possible

Track 5. Chapter 6 Self-hypnosis Script:
Sugar Avoidance

Track 6. Chapter 7 Self-hypnosis Script:
Slowing the Pace of Eating

Track 7. Chapter 8 Self-hypnosis Script:
Exercise

Track 8. Chapter 9 Self-hypnosis Script:
Changing Your Focus

Contents

Acknowledgments vii

Audio CD Contents viii

Introduction xi

How to Use the Audio CD xviii

Chapter One. Hypnosis and Self-hypnosis for Weight Loss:
Rewiring Your Brain 1

Self-hypnosis Script One: Rewiring Your Brain 14

Chapter Two. Learning to Think Differently about Losing Weight . . .21

Self-hypnosis Script Two: This Precious Moment 34

Chapter Three. This Is Not about Dieting 41

Self-hypnosis Script Three: Decision Making 56

Chapter Four. Why Do You Want to Lose Weight? 65

Self-hypnosis Script Four: Die Young as Late in Life as Possible 72

Chapter Five. Why Do You Overeat? 79

Chapter Six. Overeating Is Dangerous .95

Self-hypnosis Script Five: Sugar Avoidance 106

Chapter Seven. Thinking about Your Behavior 113

Self-hypnosis Script Six: Slowing the Pace of Eating 121

Chapter Eight. The Importance of Exercise 127

Self-hypnosis Script Seven: Exercise 138

Chapter Nine. The Body as a Pleasure Source 143

Self-hypnosis Script Eight: Changing Your Focus 151

Chapter Ten. Lifestyle Change Suggestions 157

Chapter Eleven. Menus and Recipes 177

Notes 227

References 231

About the Author 236

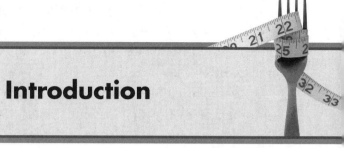

Introduction

"I've learned that you can look to people and programs for inspiration to jump-start yourself, but you have to develop a plan that will work for your life. There are no shortcuts or secrets, no magic patches or pills...You've got to love yourself and do the work it takes to sustain your most powerful engine: good health. Without it, nothing else matters."
—Oprah Winfrey

"Self-discipline burns away impurities and kindles the sparks of divinity."
—Yoga Sutras

Are you tired of not having any clothes that fit? Is being discriminated against because of your weight creating problems for you? Do you tire easily when chasing your kids or grandkids around the yard? Do you have better things to spend your money on than another fad diet book or diet pill? Do you envy people who are of average weight? Do you *never* want to diet again? If you can answer "yes" to any of these questions, keep reading.

It has been eighteen years since I introduced this weight loss program to my first patient. Since then, I have helped hundreds of people lose weight and keep it off. Most of them had tried numerous diets that failed. My program, however, motivated individuals to become responsible for their own success and to be the controller of their weight and not give up control to a pill or a fad diet. My program is not so much about eating as it is about thinking. It is about your attitude, your body, and your approach to life in general. It can instill in you a new appreciation of your body—one that allows you to embrace, value, and delight in your body even if it is not rail thin. I want you to learn to view eating and nurturing your body as a pleasurable, guilt-free endeavor, while at the same time losing weight.

And it works. My success can become your success.

There is no question in my mind that anyone who is overweight would like to lose weight. Even people who claim to be "fat and happy" deep down really do want to lose weight despite their protests to the contrary. Fear of failure, avoidance of the possible difficulty of losing weight, or rebellion against the establishment, spouse, or parents leads them to claim that they don't want to lose weight. *Think Yourself Thin* is, among other things, a compilation of experiences with many patients.

Their real-life experiences and feedback have helped me to figure out which methods really work, including hypnosis and self-hypnosis scripts.

At the end of most of the following chapters, you will find a self-hypnosis script that reinforces the concepts in that particular chapter. The self-hypnosis scripts will help you make the necessary changes by incorporating the suggestions given in the chapter at a deeper level. The included hypnosis compact disc is designed to reinforce everything that is written in this book and to put an end to your struggle to keep weight off permanently. The CD will begin to effect changes in your subconscious mind immediately, which will empower your conscious mind to change your brain, your behavior, and ultimately your life. You will want to begin listening to the hypnosis CD at least once a week as soon as you can.

Almost all of the patients I have worked with complain that they tell themselves over and over not to eat something, to stop eating when they are full, to exercise, and other such directives, but something prevents them from following their own advice. That "something" is, among other things, an area of your brain that has been strengthened as a result of giving in to cravings to overeat that are not based on hunger. My strategy begins to change that area of your brain—where those faulty cravings originate—through cognitive behavior therapy, hypnosis, self-hypnosis scripts, and much more. The suggestions on the CD and the directives in the self-hypnosis scripts actually become your own because they are, to some extent, incorporated into your mind and eventually change your brain.

I would like for you to understand on a psychological level how hypnosis works. It is important for you to know that there is no universally accepted definition of hypnosis nor is there a consensus on how it works. The hypnosis CD included here will not put you into a deep trance and many would argue that this is not possible with hypnosis. Most agree that all hypnosis is really self-hypnosis. Hypnosis is recognized worldwide as a safe and effective tool for behavior change, especially behaviors like overeating, smoking, nail biting, and other habit disorders. The hypnosis CD used in this program puts you into a deep state of relaxation in which you are highly receptive to your own thoughts. Your attention is narrowed and focused and your mind becomes quiet. In this deeply relaxed state you are more receptive to the introduction of a new thought. Your conscious mind is relaxed to the point where your subconscious mind hears the messages in a different way. Since you know that the repeated criticisms from your conscious mind have not helped you to stop overeating, the messages you need to give yourself must occur elsewhere. That place is your subconscious mind. Hypnosis is about refocusing your mind to gain greater control over your eating habits. You become so mentally focused using the positive reinforcements and guided imagery from the hypnosis that your awareness of your cravings decreases and eventually fades away. As you will learn, not only does your awareness of your cravings diminish, but the actual circuitry of your brain begins to change. That area of your brain where the cravings originate diminishes in size and activity.

This does not mean that your conscious mind is not important: there is a great deal of knowledge in this book that will be absorbed by your conscious mind and will be tremendously beneficial. It is just more important for you to learn that much of the power to help you stop overeating will come from your subconscious mind. The hypnosis CD and self-hypnosis scripts at the end of each chapter, along with many other suggestions, are going to radically change your mindset about losing weight. However, *you* will be the one who ultimately decides what works for you and what doesn't. You will determine which approaches are most effective at slimming you on the outside while simultaneously helping you to grow as a person on the inside.

This is not another diet book. If that is what you are looking for, there are hundreds available. I will explain to you in detail why the most popular diets—Atkins, Ornish, Sears (The Zone), Weight Watchers/NutriSystem–type diets—do not work long-term. Be assured that several more diet books will be published this year. There are millions of them in print right now. People continue their quest for the magic formula to help them shed unwanted pounds. Therein lies the problem, because there is no magic formula for weight loss. This book isn't about a magic formula. It is about your conscious mind, your subconscious mind, your thoughts, feelings, beliefs, attitudes, behaviors, and your relationship with your body. This book will change your approach to weight loss radically because it will begin to change your mind—and ultimately your brain.

My strategy, while certainly not easy for everyone, has the potential to end the misery for many overweight individuals and their loved ones. It is an all-encompassing strategy that incorporates many areas of your life, not just eating and exercising. I have been following my plan and monitoring patients who have been on the plan for years. Many of my patients have remained at a stable, healthy weight.

I made the decision to write this book with the intention of reaching thousands instead of just the hundreds of people who come to my office. It has become ever more disturbing for me to see people I care about become ill as a result of being overweight. It is increasingly difficult to hear their stories of suffering from heart disease, diabetes, and a whole host of debilitating conditions because they were unable to lose weight.

I was also motivated to write this book by the many patients for whom weight was not their primary problem. They would come to me with a myriad of problems, in many cases unrelated to being overweight. We would work diligently, following well-conceived and effective treatment plans. Yet, while many of their goals would be achieved, their weight problems kept them from getting well. In most cases, good mental health depends on good physical health.

It is possible that friends or family members will pick up this book in an effort to encourage someone else to lose weight. This is a situation that must be handled delicately. Pass the book on to that person, but do not push it on him. Losing weight is a personal decision and not one that can be made by someone else.

As you read this book, put yourself on the therapy couch, if you will. Try to see yourself in the examples I give and see if you can find a new approach to losing weight. It could prove a fruitful journey for you.

Congratulations on making the adult decision to *Think Yourself Thin.*

—Darcy D. Buehler, PhD

How to Use the Audio CD

Most weight-loss strategies involve dieting, in which your will is directed toward staying away from certain foods for a certain amount of time, but not about eliminating unhealthy urges altogether.

Using this CD, your will is directed toward addressing your most internal thoughts, urges, and finally, that area of your brain that generates the unhealthy cravings. With this approach you will be replacing the cravings with healthier thoughts and images and as a result will change your brain.

Your new brain circuitry will support and sometimes even initiate new urges fundamental to your new lifestyle. As you repeatedly listen to the CD and internalize the messages and make them your own, the guidance then is not from my voice, but rather deep in your own mind and the heart of direct experience.

The messages are also designed as a means of turning toward oneself with care and well-being. If you are an over-weight person, this kind of care and nurturing from yourself is a rare experience. The negative messages that you repeatedly give yourself block the much-needed inner-directed care. Messages of fear, doubt, shame, and judgment are replaced with images of confidence and psychological strength.

When you listen to the CD, you should willfully focus on the words. If your mind starts to wander—and we don't always control where our thoughts go—just gently guide your attention back to the present moment and the sound of my voice on the CD.

One of the reasons self-hypnosis is so powerful is that the pleasing images of yourself that you create in your mind produce endorphins. Endorphins are a brain chemical considered the body's natural painkiller and will replace your food urges and cravings that you used in the past to numb you to painful emotions. As your body produces these endorphins in your brain, you are less likely to have an urge for food because of the satisfied feeling you get from endorphins.

This self-hypnosis strategy begins to put your mind on what you are *for*, as opposed to what you are against. With this strategy, your emphasis is on your commitment to your body.

The eight tracks on the CD correspond to the eight self-hypnosis scripts in the book.

Choose the script that you would like to listen to, and find a comfortable place to sit or lie down. Close your eyes and spend a moment relaxing and focusing on your breathing. You may wish to scan your body, consciously relaxing your muscles, releasing any tension you may feel in your body. When you feel relaxed and focused, start the audio.

You may read through the entire book and then work your way through the CD, or you may go chapter by chapter, listening to each script as you read it in the book.

You may listen to each track as many times as you would like to. I recommend that you listen to the CD at least weekly until you reach your ideal weight. After that, you may listen whenever you wish to as a refresher.

Chapter One

Hypnosis and Self-Hypnosis for Weight Loss: Rewiring Your Brain

*"With our attention resting steadily in the present,
our bondage to past conditioning slowly dissipates."*
—Rolf Gates

The most important thing for you to learn right now is how the mind changes the brain on a physical level, and that your *will* is a physical force that can do it. When you see this, you will begin to understand why the hypnosis CD, self-hypnosis scripts, and the ideas in this book will rewire your brain and enable you to get thin and stay thin. Once you understand how this connection between your mind and your brain works, you will understand how your willful decision to change your lifestyle will enable you to overcome your ingrained, uncontrollable responses to urges to overeat or to eat unhealthy food. From the first word of this book to the last word on the hypnosis CD, the goal is to empower your mind and, ultimately, change your brain.

Your mind and your brain are not the same thing. Research has finally proven that your mind can change your brain. This is not blind faith. This is not asking you to believe that the hypnosis CD and self-hypnosis scripts themselves will change you, but the way you use them and your new way of thinking about losing weight will enable your mind to change your brain. Don't confuse the means with the end. This is about getting the right ideas into your mind so that your *will* to lose weight can alter your brain in such a way that your unwanted urges can be worked out of your brain circuitry. There is a stream of consciousness within you right now, and you need to learn to focus your attention in a way that is not fixed by your present brain state and past conditioning. This is the heart of this book—to teach you to focus your attention in a way that is not determined by previous behavior and thought patterns. Your *will*, strengthened by self-hypnosis and reinforced by your new way of thinking, will work to undo the tangle of conditioning that has accumulated, possibly for years, to create your present brain state and cause you to overeat. The hypnosis CD and the self-hypnosis scripts contain the specific knowledge you need and are written in such a way that they will empower your mind to change your brain.

You must understand that your will is a physical force. It is not only a thought, as was once believed, but it is also a focusing of your attention, and it has been proven to exist in the physical world as a force. Brain imaging technology proves that will generates a force, and that the force can effect physical changes in the brain, such as which areas of the brain show activity with certain urges. Through exerting your will, you can literally rewire areas of the brain that determine and generate the urges regarding food and eating habits. Brain change has been proven to occur in obsessive-compulsive disorder (OCD) patients with just ten weeks of *self-directed* cognitive behavior therapy. In the opinion of this author, overeating is a compulsive behavior, and if you have had the willpower to go on a diet for three months, then you can easily work through this program, which combines self-directed cognitive behavior therapy with self-hypnosis and much more to help you change your brain, your behavior, and ultimately your life.

The good news is that compulsive overeating is not nearly as severe a brain imbalance as actual OCD. Obsessive-compulsive disordered individuals were probably born with their disorder. You were not born a compulsive overeater. Most likely you can remember a time before you obsessed about food. This was a time when you listened to your body and ate only when you received healthy signals to eat as a result of your body needing food for sustenance. The circuits in your brain that misfire to give you the urge to overeat are probably not very well-developed, but are a result of repeatedly giving in to these urges. Because your urges are not well-developed, they are more easily changed.

Regardless of their severity, these urges need to be changed, and the key is the force of your will. In order to understand the concept of will, you need to consider the mind separately from the brain. For years, many in the scientific community have considered the brain to be responsible for behavior and have not given the role of the mind due credit. The mind may depend on the brain for its expression, but many aspects of the mind occur independently of the brain.

When I refer to the brain, I'm talking about actual brain matter: the physical qualities of the organ. Mind is much more than gray matter. Mind is our attention, our felt inner awareness, our consciousness, and much more. Research is proving that the mind influences the brain, and the structure of the brain can, as a matter of fact, be changed with repeated focus of your will.

The definition of "will" probably dates back to 1890, when William James determined it to "prolong a stay in consciousness of innumerable ideas which else would fade away more quickly." American Heritage Dictionary defines "will" as "the mental faculty by which one deliberately chooses or decides upon a course of action." When you realize that will is now recognized in science as a physical force, you can see that the "prolonged stay in consciousness" James referred to is, in fact, a course of action. The hypnosis CD, the self-hypnosis scripts, and the new way of thinking about weight loss presented in this book enable you to create and imprint certain ideas in a prolonged stay of consciousness in your mind, and the resulting physical action of your will on the brain causes it to change. The overall result is a reduction of activity in the area of your brain where unhealthy food urges occur. That course of action will dramatically reduce your unhealthy urges to overeat.

Remember, if you've had the willpower to go on a diet for three months, then you have the willpower to work through this program, practice the self-hypnosis scripts, listen to the CD, change the way you think, and make some permanent changes regarding your behavior and your weight. The brain changes in OCD patients have been demonstrated in just ten weeks of self-directed therapy. With this program, you have much more at your disposal than just self-directed therapy.

For eighteen years, I have had many, many patients lose weight with the use of hypnosis, self-hypnosis, and learning to think themselves thin. I knew that it worked, and now I am aware of the physical mechanism within the brain that explains why it works in the long run. My patients lost weight and kept it off because they were changing the circuitry of their brains. Jeffrey M. Schwartz, MD, author of *Brain Lock, The Mind and the Brain* and *Dear Patrick: Letters to a Young Man*, led the research at UCLA, which documented, in his own words: "cognitive-behavior therapy—or, indeed, any psychiatric treatment that did not rely on drugs—has the power to change brain chemistry in a well-identified brain circuit...Self-directed therapy had dramatically and significantly altered brain function."

The following images illustrate the brain changes that occurred as a result of self-directed cognitive therapy.

location where brain slice is taken

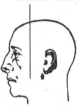

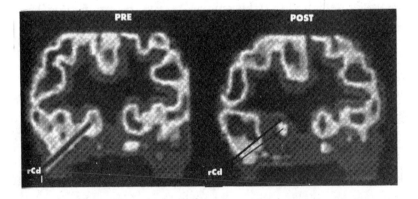

PET (positron emission tomography) scans of a patient with OCD, before and after two months of therapy. The decrease in energy is easy to see in the right caudate (rCd)—the Post image (right) is much smaller.

Copyright 1996, *Archives of General Psychiatry*, February 1996, pages 109–113. Reprinted by permission. Also appeared in *The Mind and the Brain*, page 89; and in *Brain Lock*, page 59.

There is plenty of data from brain imaging technology to support the idea that this sort of self-directed therapy causes significant changes in brain circuitry. Functional magnetic resonance imaging (fMRI) of the brain has illustrated and proven that this has happened with OCD patients. It was the repeated focus of their will—away from the urges—that caused the change. Dr. Jeffrey M. Schwartz provided the following comment for *Think Yourself Thin*: "Concerning the problem of obesity, perhaps our main impediment to developing a proper and healthy awareness of the sense of satiety [fullness] is that we have been indoctrinated as a culture to experience our bodily feelings solely as products of brain machinery, and therefore out of our control. Now we know that this is false. There is a lot we can do with our mental efforts to alter the machinery of the brain. We now know that cognitive training empowers us to alter the hunger mechanism of the brain so that we can effectively prevent ourselves from habitual and mindless overeating."

Dr. Schwartz confirms that the ideas presented in this book have the potential to provide us with an entirely new and different way of approaching weight loss. He agrees that we have much at our disposal to help us begin responding differently to our urges to overeat. We are no longer held prisoner to an urge to overeat when in fact we are not hungry.

With my patients, hypnosis, self-hypnosis, and learning to think differently provided the method for them to focus their will away from their desire to overeat. It worked. Repeated successes with my patients have shown that the methods in this book can end the diet roller-coaster forever.

You can begin right now to incorporate the self-hypnosis scripts as you read this book and listen to the CD to begin changing your brain. You've just seen how the brain changes—now you are ready to see how this strategy will help you lose weight.

You must begin to see your urges to overeat in a new way. If you begin to see your urges as something that is occurring within your brain, it will help you to distance yourself from them. *You are not your urges.* It is not that you are a weak, undisciplined loser, as I have heard some patients call themselves, but the fact that over the years your brain has sent many faulty messages. You have gradually changed the structure of your brain by giving in to those messages repeatedly. A non-judgmental, non-critical view of the messages creates a very different emotional reaction. It also helps to purposefully shift away from identifying so closely with intrusive thoughts and urges to overeat. *You are not these intrusive thoughts.* Viewing your urges and thoughts from this perspective prevents you from being hypercritical of yourself because you have them. By telling yourself repeatedly that the urges are faulty messages from your brain, you can begin to react to them with a new and different mindset. You will do this by using the hypnosis CD and self-hypnosis scripts, which will help you to be more mindful and strengthen the effort of your will. You will, with time, be able to put mental space between your will and the unwanted urges—no more excuses that you don't have the willpower. You *do* have the willpower; you have just allowed faulty brain circuitry to overpower your will.

If you can view your thoughts and urges simply as faulty brain circuitry, you will be less likely to judge yourself for having them and less likely to give in to them. For example, you say to yourself, "This desire for sugar reflects a malfunction of my brain, and not a real need to put food into my mouth, especially since I just ate one hour ago and my stomach is still full." Or, "This urge for a second helping is false and misleading because I am now comfortably full." One of my patients said that she likes to think of the urges like spam email that appears on her computer. She simply presses the delete button to rid herself of them. With continued effort, it will begin to seem that easy to refute your urges.

You will see that the self-hypnosis program will enable you to overcome your urges to overeat. You will not necessarily ignore the urges; you will acknowledge them, remember they are faulty brain messages, and replace them—mindfully and willfully—with positive thoughts and images. The faulty messages will simply fade away.

This new mode of thinking is one of the primary cognitive training strategies you will use. Over and over, you will refuse to accept food cravings at face value. By saying no to these cravings, you begin to see that the urges to keep eating when you are full or to eat foods that are unhealthy are inherently false and misleading.

Repeatedly relabeling these urges as false will begin to diminish the unpleasant feeling you get from them significantly. You will gradually begin to feel a greater sense of control because, by repeatedly refuting these cravings, your mind actually changes the amount of energy occurring in that area of the brain where the cravings originate. You begin to feel a sense of freedom because you are no longer controlled by your urges.

This strategy also slows down the process, allowing you to see how things work. Instead of being swept away by old patterns, you have a choice between blind reaction and a considered, creative response. This prevents semiconscious eating, which inevitably leads to mistakes.

Compare this approach to weight loss with dieting. With dieting, you are told to eat different foods for a while, but your urges for unhealthy foods are still there. Your will is directed toward staying on the diet, rather than addressing your most internal thoughts, urges, and ultimately brain chemistry. You are still feeding the urges, so they will not fade away. The purpose of this approach is to replace unhealthy urges with new thoughts and habits, which will change your brain, and result in healthier urges that support your new lifestyle.

The problem is not so much that you need to be told what to eat and what not to eat; the bigger problem is how you deal with your urges. Unlike diet books, this book addresses those urges and provides a specific strategy. If you learn to respond differently to your urges, you can succeed in permanent weight loss.

The mental process you are about to embark upon will, over time, embed new thoughts into the brain. Once this is done, the new thoughts and urges will outweigh the old—and you will *stay* thin. Your brain circuitry will now support—and sometimes even initiate—the urges fundamental to your new healthy lifestyle.

At the end of most of the chapters, I have included a self-hypnosis script to help you internalize and incorporate the suggestions of that chapter into your lifestyle. As you repeat the scripts several times, you internalize them and make them your own. The guidance, then, is not from the pages or my voice, but rather from deep within your own mind and the heart of your direct experience. The intention of the hypnosis CD and self-hypnosis scripts is to internalize or program certain insights into your mind, gradually deepen your commitment to your lifestyle changes, and ultimately change your brain. The self-hypnosis practice enhances your ability to focus your attention away from otherwise determined mental habits. As you repeatedly listen to each segment, you will become strengthened in your resolve to lose weight and make good decisions regarding your eating.

The practice of self-hypnosis is also a means of focusing upon oneself with care and well-being. If you are overweight, this kind of care and nurturing from yourself is a rare experience. The negative messages that you give yourself repeatedly impede much-needed, inner-directed care. However, when you nurture yourself messages of fear, doubt, shame, and judgment are replaced with images of confidence and psychological strength. Your mind is focused all too often on negative messages, or you are bombarding yourself with moralistic pronouncements, neither of which contribute to the new mindset you will need to lose weight.

When you listen to the hypnosis CD or read the self-hypnosis scripts, you are not just *reading* them, you must focus willfully on the words. It is critical to this program that the words are read *mindfully*, with focused attention. As noted at the beginning of the chapter, Rolf Gates said, "With our attention resting steadily in the present, our bondage to past conditioning slowly dissipates." This is the state of mind you need to be in while you listen to the CD or read the self-hypnosis scripts. If your mind begins to wander—and we don't always control where our thoughts go—you must learn to guide your attention gently back to the present moment and the sound of my voice or the printed word.

Each self-hypnosis segment begins with instructions to concentrate on your breathing and relax your body. You will be asked to maintain a rhythmic, even breathing cadence as you read the script. Breathing in this manner results in relaxation and tension reduction. You will read the self-hypnosis script silently or aloud, have someone read it to you, or make a recording of it and listen to it in your own voice. The hypnosis CD provides extended versions of each segment. You will use both methods, but with the hypnosis CD, your eyes will be closed, allowing you to go deeper into self-hypnosis and enhance your visualization.

One reason the hypnosis CD and self-hypnosis scripts are so powerful is because the pleasing images you will be asked to create in your mind produce the brain chemical endorphin. Endorphins are associated with pleasure and are the body's natural painkillers. Endorphins will replace food urges that you have used in the past to numb you from the inevitable pain of being human. As your body produces these in your brain, you are less likely to have an urge for food because of the satisfied feeling you get from the endorphins.

In whatever way you choose to use the self-hypnosis scripts, it is important to get yourself into a relaxed, meditative frame of mind. Start by focusing on your breathing. Do not alter the natural rhythm of your breathing; just begin to notice the rising and falling of the chest, the sensation of the inhalation and exhalation on the supple tissue of your nostrils. You may want to concentrate on the rhythm of your heartbeat. Continue the relaxed, rhythmic breathing for two to three minutes before you read the self-hypnosis script, and maintain that rhythm throughout. On the hypnosis CD, you will be given specific instructions to help you become relaxed.

It is important to attend mindfully to each word you read or hear. When you read the self-hypnosis scripts, read them at a slower pace than you normally read. When you begin to visualize (and, even if you read, you will eventually visualize what you have read with your eyes closed), do not think of visualizing with your eyes. Rather, imagine the visualizations appearing within the mind in its own space. You will see yourself in the visualizations within your mind. It is usually recommended that you focus on a point between and just above the eyes, the so-called "third eye." Imagine that you are looking at this point from a distance a little further back inside your head.

I am now going to introduce you to an actual self-hypnosis script. Remember that, even though initially you will read the script, eventually you will visualize what you have read with your eyes closed. While you are listening to the hypnosis CD, you want to have your eyes closed. Then, throughout your day, you will occasionally visualize yourself making successful choices as suggested by the CD and scripts. It will be helpful to read the scripts or listen to the CD over and over. Depending on your own personal needs, you can choose which script suits you at any given time. Read them at least several times per week. Remember, you are imprinting your brain with these thoughts, and you need to read them often enough for them to become part of you.

Also, notice that the scripts are written in the second person. This is because the first few times you read them, they need to come to you from an encouraging and instructional standpoint. Once you feel as though you've received enough encouragement and instruction and feel enough self-confidence, I suggest that you translate them into the first person and read them that way ("I" rather than "you").

Self-hypnosis Script One:
Rewiring Your Brain

In this chapter you have learned that the brain sends faulty messages to your mind and that you behave (i.e., eat) according to those faulty messages. You also learned that you can change the circuitry of your brain by refuting these faulty messages over and over again. This session is designed to help you change your thinking and, ultimately, the circuitry of your brain.

In a nice, comfortable position, begin to concentrate on your steady, even breathing.

Begin to clear your mind of all the thoughts of your day and bring your attention to your body as it begins to relax. Notice any tightness or tension leaving your body.

Inhale and exhale, naturally and rhythmically.

Inhale—expand; exhale—release.

Let your body sink deeper and deeper into the cushions beneath you as you become more and more relaxed.

Slowly, gradually, and comfortably, noticing the rising and falling of your chest, you are becoming more relaxed.

In a pleasant state of relaxation, you are reading the printed words in front of you and becoming more and more relaxed.

You are going to focus your attention on the suggestions given to you that are acceptable to you.

Anytime your mind wanders, you will gently bring your attention back to these words in front of you.

With the strength of your will and the power of your mind, you are going to begin making changes in your eating behavior.

Not because I am telling you, but because of the strength of your mind, you are going to begin changing your brain and your eating behavior.

You are going to become stronger in your resolve to lose weight consistently and permanently.

Begin seeing yourself at your ideal weight and feeling very good about yourself.

You are feeling very excited to have found a new strategy to lose weight permanently and consistently.

This strategy will help you to put your mind on what you are for—healthy weight loss—rather than what you are against.

That's right: you will begin to believe that you can—and will—lose weight, and that you will finally be able to say "no" to unhealthy urges to eat.

Begin to visualize yourself in those situations in which you have found yourself confronted with difficult food choices.

See yourself at home, at work, out visiting family and friends, or out at your favorite restaurant. Notice how good you are feeling.

Notice that your brain is urging you to eat something when you are already full or something that is no longer part of your new lifestyle.

Begin to notice the interchange going on in your thinking system.

Take note of the faulty message that is telling you to eat when you know that you are not hungry, or the message urging you to eat something that no longer fits into your lifestyle.

Be very aware of the pleasant, full feeling in your stomach.

You might also be aware at other times that you are not full, but that you will be eating in a couple of hours and that it is your desire to be pleasantly hungry when it is time to eat.

Be very clear in your mind that these false messages are just that: faulty messages based on old-fashioned, worn-out habits that have negatively affected your life.

Be clear in your mind that there is no need to respond to the message, no reason to allow yourself to cave in to these faulty messages, no need to eat when you are not hungry.

Your urges are nothing more than faulty messages from your brain. You are learning to recognize a false message and simply say no to urges.

You can and you will refuse to give in to these urges and recognize them as false.

That's right, you can refuse to accept the messages and see them as nothing more than a poor attempt by your brain to control your behavior.

The pesky messages from your brain will no longer control what you eat. You will control what goes into your mouth and feel very good about it.

Slowly, but surely, your mind can begin to change the structure of your brain, and as the structure of your brain changes, the urges diminish.

You see yourself refuting the negative messages that you are receiving from your brain over and over again—and gradually changing the structure of your brain.

That's right, the more often you say no to unhealthy food urges, the easier it becomes.

More and more, you will not allow yourself to eat based on these distorted messages when you know that you are not really hungry.

The urges and desires based on false messages are not the problem. Allowing yourself to be controlled by them is the problem, and you will no longer be controlled by faulty messages.

Very soon, you will begin to enjoy the relief of having the desires pass and of no longer being harassed by them.

Totally relaxed and calm, begin to visualize yourself refuting these false messages over and over, feeling stronger and stronger, having no desire to give in to these distorted messages.

That's right—you are feeling very strong, and having no desire to give in to the faulty messages.

You see yourself in many situations, and, if at any time you receive one of these false messages, you see yourself feeling very excited about how well you are able to refute the message and not give into it.

That's right, you see yourself taking two or three deep breaths, giving yourself the time you need to refute the message.

As you inhale, you imagine confidence welling up in your chest—you feel the psychological strength coursing through your body and your brain.

Over and over, you are able to refute these distorted messages. Each time you see yourself refuting the message, you know that your mind is, in fact, changing your brain.

You are strengthening the neural pathways that help you say "no" to false messages.

You are very excited about knowing that the desires are empty, and that even though the desire may pull, it is really empty.

Your brain, in a very interesting way, is going to begin working for you rather than against you.

Your new brain circuitry, in a very interesting way, is going to gain strength each time you refute one of those old-fashioned, embarrassing urges.

It will begin to feel natural to refute those messages and maintain the lifestyle changes you have made.

That's right, each time that you redefine an urge as a misfire from your brain, the old-fashioned messages will become weaker and your lifestyle changes will become stronger.

You can almost feel the strength and excitement in your heart center as you develop and maintain a healthy lifestyle.

Your mind can—and will—change the nature of your brain as it becomes easier and easier to maintain your lifestyle changes.

You are feeling very excited about finally finding a strategy to help you deal with those unwanted urges to overeat.

Your urges to overeat are diminishing, and your new lifestyle is becoming stronger.

You feel very good about yourself and your decision to *think yourself thin*.

Chapter Two

Learning to Think Differently about Losing Weight

*"Our THOUGHTS, our words, our deeds
are threads of the net we throw around ourselves."*
—Swami Vivekanada

I will lose weight. I can control what I put into my mouth. I cannot wait to begin losing weight. I am excited about being free of harmful eating habits. I will lose weight and keep it off this time. I will adjust happily to a more slender form. Is this the kind of thinking that you use when you prepare yourself to lose weight?

Or is your thinking more along these lines: *I hope I can lose weight this time. I've failed to lose weight with so many diets. No diet has ever really worked for me. I wonder if this program will fail. I'll try, but I'm pretty skeptical about it working. I'm not sure I can really lose weight. My eating habits are so deeply ingrained that I'm not sure anything will ever work for me. I've tried to lose weight so many times that I feel pretty discouraged about trying again.* Is this the kind of self-talk you use as you prepare to go on a diet?

As an experiment, I would like for you to reread the italicized sentences in the first and second paragraphs. See if the two paragraphs invoke different emotional responses for you. My hunch is—and research suggests—that the first paragraph will actually leave you feeling more confident that you will lose weight.

As a therapist, I use a technique called cognitive restructuring with patients with all types of psychological problems. Cognitive restructuring really means changing your thinking and suggests that what you think and the things you tell yourself create the way you feel to a great extent. You can change the way you feel about a situation by changing the way you think about it. You can probably think of many situations in which two individuals shared the same experience and had very different reactions. This is largely because their thoughts about the situation were so different. It is not necessarily the situation that causes you to feel a certain way, but, rather, how you think about it. We also know that the way we feel influences the way we behave.

Cognitive restructuring creates a positive mindset that often supersedes the need to refute negative messages and urges from your brain. If you can develop a strong belief in your ability to lose weight, you are already ahead of the game, as you will have significantly fewer urges to overeat in the first place.

A good example, though unrelated to losing weight, may help you understand the benefits of restructuring your cognitions and the effect your thinking has on your feelings and behaviors. A patient of mine named LuAnn told me about walking into work one day as one of her colleagues rushed by her in the hall, barely acknowledging her presence. She initially thought about the experience with her colleague from the following perspective:

Scenario #1: "Wow, Ashley was really unfriendly! I wonder what I did to make her mad at me. I wonder why she snubbed me like that." With this sort of thinking, you may end up feeling bad about yourself. However, after LuAnn remembered her cognitive therapy work, she thought about it from the following perspective.

Scenario #2: "Wow, Ashley was really in a big hurry! She's usually pretty busy. I'll have to catch up with her later today and find out what was going on." Ashley was as friendly as usual when LuAnn met her later in the day. LuAnn found out during the conversation that Ashley was rushing to a very important meeting early that morning, had a lot on her mind, and was running late. Thinking about the encounter from a scenario #2 perspective saved LuAnn a lot of anguish.

Scenario #1 is an example of a commonly used cognitive distortion called "personalization." Personalization occurs when you see yourself as the cause of some external negative event (being ignored) for which, in fact, you were not responsible.

As you read this book, you will begin to change the way you think about losing weight. You will start believing that you can and will lose weight. I have had zero patients in fifteen years who had not tried to lose weight previously. The majority had tried several diets. It is the history of failure, and fear of future failure, that keep most people thinking that they cannot lose weight. Most of my patients have tried the popular diets and procedures, including Weight Watchers, NutriSystem, Atkins, TOPS (Take off Pounds Sensibly), stomach stapling, and more. By the time someone gets to my office, after having failed on several of these programs, they are not only extremely discouraged, but also fairly convinced that they cannot lose weight. Remember, it is your failure history and your belief that you will fail again that gets in the way of your weight loss. It has very little to do with the present. What occurred in the past actually has nothing to do with your current effort to lose weight. You can and will put your past failures behind you once and for all.

Self-efficacy—the belief that you will be successful—is an extremely important factor in weight loss. It is one of the best predictors of behavior change. Researchers have found that your belief that you can accomplish something leads to a greater likelihood of success. There are a number of strategies in my program that will help you to lose weight, but even those strategies won't *work unless you believe you can do it.*

How do you change your thinking and beliefs about your ability to lose weight? You change your self-talk. Self-talk is exactly what it sounds like: talking to yourself. Most people carry on a dialogue within their own mind most of the time, anyway. I am telling you that you can learn to control your self-talk and use it to help you lose weight. The first step in changing your thinking is to write down your positive self-talk statements. Here are some examples. After you read them, write down your own list, using some or all of these examples, as well as some of your own.

1. I will lose weight.
2. I am looking forward to losing weight.
3. I am confident that I will lose weight.
4. Food will never again control my life.
5. I am excited about giving up my old eating habits.
6. I have the willpower to control my eating.
7. I will happily change my lifestyle.
8. I will change my identity from overeater to healthy eater.
9. I will control the food I put in my mouth.
10. Past failures to lose weight will not interfere with my current success.

As you prepare to change your lifestyle, you will spend a little time each day looking over your personal self-talk statements. You will be encouraged by how these positive statements will gradually begin to change the way you feel about losing weight. You will gradually gain healthy control over your eating.

Number nine on the above positive self-talk list refers to gaining control over what you put in your mouth. I'd like you to stop reading for a few minutes and think of those things in your life over which you have complete control.

Did you think about them? My guess is that you probably came up with very few things. Even if you live by yourself, work by yourself, and lead a very solitary existence, there are still very few things over which you have complete control. Our mobile, interactive society contains many variables and entities that regularly impinge upon our lives and choices.

Eating is one thing over which, in reality, you have complete control. There are very few things over which you have more control than what goes into your mouth. You're going to learn how to exercise that control.

You will begin to think differently about the concept of effort. Once you begin to believe in yourself and your ability to lose weight, it is time to apply the necessary effort and energy. Anything you have ever accomplished in your life has happened because you put forth effort. You understand effort, because you have exerted effort many times in your life. No doubt there have been times that you had to dig in and do something extra to sustain your effort *en route* to accomplishment.

I want you to begin to think about effort as occurring in three basic stages. You will persevere through all three stages until maintaining your healthy weight will begin to feel like second nature to you. It will begin to feel as if the energy generated from your effort continually grows and feeds on itself. Because of the changes you are making in your brain, your effort is something you know you can sustain.

The first stage is the launching, or preliminary, effort. This stage involves the courage and willingness to begin a program. You are reading this book, so you are clearly in the first stage. If you have ever dieted, you have probably navigated this stage and actually lost some weight. In fact, it is theorized that it is the initial success at this stage that causes compulsive dieters to try each new fad diet that comes out. The memory of this success is more salient than the ensuing failure to maintain the lost weight.

The second stage is the transcending effort, which requires you to be diligent enough not to be dissuaded or to falter when things become more difficult. What most often happens at this stage is that the body's natural adjustment to different eating habits causes the weight loss to slow down and plateau. There may actually be brief periods during which no weight is lost at all. When the weight does not come off as quickly as it did at the outset of your lifestyle changes, it is often misinterpreted as exhaustion of effort. Trust yourself and your level of effort. Do not get discouraged and think that all is lost because you are not losing weight quickly. Even if you have a minor relapse, under-stand that it is part of the journey to eventual permanent weight loss. My hope is that, because you do not have unrealistic expectations, you will not get discouraged when the weight loss inevitably slows down.

If you can persevere through this stage and make it to the progressive, or developed, effort (the third stage), you will arrive at a quality of energy that does not decrease or stagnate. When you sustain your effort at this stage, you will feel an energy level that seems to grow in power, eventually leading to a sense of freedom. For example, you may go twenty-five days without a snack at three o'clock in the afternoon because you have decided that it no longer fits your lifestyle, and there is no way on the twenty-sixth day that you are going to have a snack at three o'clock. In fact, you will have very little desire for that snack and may not even think about it or experience the urge to have it. Because of the changes in your brain, you are more likely to make it to this stage and stay there forever.

Changing your identity is another strategy that will help you begin to think differently about losing weight. We have many identities: parent, spouse, psychologist, teacher, runner, overeater, and so on. When you have tried to lose weight in the past, you have probably often felt deprived when you had to give up some of your favorite foods and decrease the quantity you were eating. The reason you felt deprived was because you had not made a shift in your identity. You were continuing to maintain identities such as overeater, junk-food eater, or food addict. All of these negative identities perpetuate a belief system that contributes to low self-esteem, feelings of deprivation, and overeating.

Instead of thinking of yourself as being deprived, you will begin to think of losing weight as something you are doing for yourself—something you are doing out of respect for your body. You will add healthy eater to your list of identities. You are choosing health over premature death from obesity. It eventually will be like liberating yourself. You will be free to choose. You will no longer be bound or trapped by a habit and negative identity that prevent you from choosing. Few people would choose consciously to kill themselves because of obesity.

You need to ask yourself, "Am I in favor of living?" If you are not in favor of living, then you might as well continue to overeat. My hunch is that the idea of living is still something that interests you. If this is the case, then it is your duty to give up your unhealthy habit of overeating and treat your body in a manner that reflects your interest in living. You must begin to respect and protect your body.

Another reason people have a difficult time losing weight is that they are constantly telling themselves, "Don't eat." That is like telling yourself, "Don't swallow" or "Don't think of an orange hippopotamus." Odds are, you will think about nothing but that orange hippopotamus. Free, independent people don't like to be told "don't." You are more likely to change your behavior on the basis of something you are for, rather than something you are against. You are in favor of showing respect for and protecting your body instead of having to tell yourself "don't." The emphasis is upon your commitment to respect and protect your body.

Many of my weight-loss patients have come to see food as an agent of comfort, almost like a friend. Unfortunately, it is a deadly friend. When they feel depressed, anxious, betrayed, bored, or discouraged, they turn to food. Much like a good friend or social support, food serves as a buffer against acknowledging these feelings. At this point, I explain to them that they need to say goodbye to food as they now see it (i.e., as a comfort or reward). This process of saying goodbye is almost a form of grieving. It is much easier to let go of someone or something when you have grieved appropriately and said goodbye.

That's what J. Anderson did in her book *A Year by the Sea*, when she explained, "Grief is the partner of change." She goes on to say, "I no longer intend to hide my feelings [e.g., grief] or inspirations in fat. I want to stand whole in my skin and fly. I'm in a race against time. I need my body to catch up with all of me to test my will and endurance. My body became a stranger I chose not to know."

Has your body become a stranger to you? If you are overeating and unhealthy, you are not embracing your physical self and experiencing your body as a source of pleasure. Rather, your body may be something you loathe, a source of shame and pain. In chapter 11, I will discuss your body as a source of pleasure.

I realize that this grieving may sound a little corny, but I have actually seen patients shed tears at the point in the session when they begin to realize that their relationship with food must change. I don't expect you to perform an elaborate grieving ceremony, but some sort of acknowledgment that you will change your relationship with food can help you to avoid old, unhealthy eating habits. We are a culture obsessed with consumption as a source of "completion." This consumption may be of material goods or food; no matter what the case may be, none of these entities can ever be your agent of completion.

As you know, thinking differently about cravings will help you lose weight. It is important to acknowledge the bodily sensations of hunger and fullness. Acknowledging and responding appropriately to these sensations is a lifestyle change that will help you shed many of those unwanted pounds.

✶ Cravings may not always be equated or associated with the sensation of hunger. If you think of these sensations as one and the same, it may be very difficult to lose weight. The mindset for many is that cravings and eating urges occur only because of physical withdrawal or when signals from your body tell you that you need to eat. I don't believe that this is always true. In fact, I believe that it is often very far from the truth. Many urges or hunger pangs are triggered by situations and circumstances completely unrelated to physical hunger. These pangs may be related to a certain time of day (such as when your children come home from school), an individual in your life, a type of feeling, or a distant memory. As you learned in chapter 1, cravings or urges are really just learned, conditioned responses that, over time, result in faulty brain messages. You are going to learn to distinguish between cravings that are a result of actual hunger and those that are faulty brain messages. If you acknowledge this difference, you can use the hypnosis CD, self-hypnosis scripts, and your new way of thinking to weaken the faulty messages. They will become weaker and weaker until, eventually, they go away completely. In chapter 5, you will learn to identify sensations associated with actual food hunger.

Most people fear that unless something is eaten, the craving will not go away. In reality, most non-hunger-based cravings are brief. This is when using cognitive restructuring is very important. You must learn to think differently about your "craving." Over time, you will weaken—and ultimately extinguish—these cravings.

Something else to remember when responding to a craving is to remain in the present moment. People often sabotage their lifestyle changes by projecting themselves into the future. If you stay in the present moment, you probably know that you can resist a current craving. The problem arises when you say to yourself, "Six hours, three days, or two weeks from now there is no way I'll be able to maintain these lifestyles changes. There is no way I'll be able to continue avoiding French fries or chocolate."

Not only is negative self-talk at work in this example, but the present has been abandoned completely for an ambiguous future moment. It is also common to allow the memory of past failures to creep in when experiencing cravings. The past is gone. Let go of it. It has nothing to do with your current weight loss regimen. This strategy is completely different from anything you have tried in the past, and what happened in the past has nothing to do with what you are doing now.

Sylvia Boorstein writes extensively about mindfulness and paying attention as the path to the end of suffering. In her book, *Pay Attention for Goodness Sake*, she writes eloquently about dealing with desires and staying in the moment:

> "I need to keep discovering that the pain of the struggle is greater than the pain of the desire. If I develop the habit of restraining myself, I'll enjoy the relief of feeling desires pass, and I'll remember that desires are not the problem. Feeling pushed around by them is. I'll continue to have desires of course, because I am alive, but they'll be more modest in their demands."

This may be helpful to you in learning to think differently about your craving for food. Humans truly have a powerful gift: the capacity for restraint. You will, of course, experience the tension of desire occasionally, but it will always pass. In the words of Sylvia Boorstein, it passes "not because I have willed it away, talked myself out of it, or even promised it for later, but just because it passes, like everything else. Remember, it's not about becoming stoic. It's about becoming intimate with the nature of desire itself. Desire pulls so hard it's surprising to find that it's empty." Although Ms. Boorstein says that desires pass "not because I have willed it away," you are learning that one of the primary strategies for losing weight is literally to diminish desire through the use of your will. Her point—that desires will pass—is important, whether through the use of your will (as described in this book), or the understanding that the nature of desire is ultimately empty, or, simply, that all things change. As you will find, your response to desires can change.

Research indicates that anticipated overeating actually leads to future overeating. This makes it all the more important to stay in the moment and not think about future situations in which you may be tempted to overeat.

Naomi, a patient, recently told me how this way of thinking really helped her. She works as a data entry specialist out of her home and goes to lunch on a regular basis with a group of friends, most of whom have unhealthy eating habits. The day before she was to go out with them, she was getting ready to fix her lunch at home. She was trying to decide what to eat and the thought entered her mind that tomorrow was her lunch date with her friends. She knew that she would be tempted to order something unhealthy. From that thought came an impulse to eat something unhealthy because she would probably blow it tomorrow, anyway. Then, she remembered my instructions about staying in the moment. Naomi put the hot dogs back into the refrigerator and had a salad and whole wheat crackers instead. She stayed in the present moment and reported that she was also able to eat healthily with her friends the next day.

You must approach this intended lifestyle change with a completely new thought process. I personally like Julia Childs's comment: "Life itself is the best binge." Start thinking that bingeing on life will be a better alternative to food. You can be satisfied with life and stop substituting food for your source of meaning and pleasure.

Self-hypnosis Script Two:
This Precious Moment

This segment is designed to help you stay in the moment in order to enhance your ability to avoid giving in to your craving. Learning to stay in the moment will also contribute to a better sense of well-being in your life in general.

Find a nice, comfortable position, and begin to focus on the rhythm of your breathing.

Practice natural, rhythmic inhalation and exhalation.

Begin to clear your mind of all the thoughts of your day.

Simply become aware of your breathing and the rhythm of your heartbeat.

Notice how good you feel right here, right now, in this precious moment.

Faced with the desire to give up this precious moment for some unknowable future or some memory from your past, just relax and bring your attention back to your breath.

We don't know about the future and the past is gone, so all we really have is this precious moment.

You will find yourself in many situations in which your natural inclination is to begin thinking about the future or the past and to begin planning, rehearsing, dreaming, or worrying.

When confronted with a decision about how you want to treat your body, stay right here, right now.

You know that, in this precious moment, right now, you can treat your body in a very healthy and wise manner.

In this precious moment, you are just fine, and you have no need to abandon your healthy lifestyle.

You will not allow yourself to be afraid of a time tomorrow, or next week, or next month, when a difficult food choice may arise.

Nor will you allow yourself to think back to last week, last month, or last year, when food choices were difficult for you.

Whether you are planning dinner out with your friends, anticipating an upcoming vacation, or looking forward to the next holiday, you will stay right here, right now, and make the right decision for your body.

It is easier, right here, right now, to give up an unhealthy food than to think about giving it up for the rest of your life.

You are learning, minute-by-minute, to let go of your fears and your desires and become free of unhealthy urges.

You are not going to worry about tomorrow, next week, or next year. Only right now, in the present, can you say "no" to unhealthy messages from your brain to indulge in unhealthy food.

Right here, right now, you are beginning to believe in your ability to make the right decision, and each minute that you believe in yourself, your capacity to make the right decisions grows.

You begin to believe that staying with this precious moment will make healthy choices easier.

You will find that any urges to overeat will grow steadily and markedly less, and will soon disappear almost completely.

You will have minor urges to overeat, but you will begin responding very differently to them. Only right now can you respond to these urges. You will respond now with no preoccupation with the past or apprehension about the future.

You will say "no" to urges—and they will go away.

You will remember these words and images from time to time. And in a very interesting way, the urges will subside.

Yes, steadily and markedly, the desire to overeat will become totally and completely within your power, rather than under the control of some pesky message from your brain.

That's right. Each right decision in this moment will make your next decision easier.

The past is gone and you cannot predict the future, so you have only this precious moment in which to make healthy choices.

And, in this precious moment, you know that you can make the right choice.

You will not allow yourself to abandon this precious moment and indulge in unhealthy eating because of a past failure or a fear of the future.

You are feeling very good about yourself and your ability to stay in the moment and make the right choice for your body.

As you learn to stay more in the present and maintain awareness of what is happening right here, right now, you will not allow yourself to indulge in past eating habits.

Remember, it is your memory of past failures and your fear of future temptation that will sabotage your lifestyle changes, and by maintaining moment-to-moment awareness, you will not allow yourself to indulge.

With your thoughts resting steadily in this moment more and more, you will find the healthy choices becoming easier and easier.

Just take a nice, deep breath and feel the confidence welling up in your chest. Take another deep breath as you feel the psychological strength coursing through your veins.

In this precious moment, you see yourself making good choices and reinforcing your new, healthy lifestyle.

This is the second of eight self-hypnosis scripts that will appear in this book. You may want to reread it a few times before going on to the next chapter. I also encourage you to come back and read it from time to time. The more you read it, as Stephen Levine says, the more it "becomes your own" and the more strongly the insights become internalized. Similarly, if you listen to the CD, the more you listen, the more strongly the messages become yours.

Chapter Three

This Is Not about Dieting

*"Dieting is a notoriously ineffective means
of achieving weight loss."*
—T. Heatherton

Rebecca, a very attractive, middle-aged woman, sat in my waiting room with a very sad look on her face. She had recently discovered that, as a result of taking fen-phen, a popular diet drug in the nineties, she had developed heart valve disease. This was after she had failed to lose weight on several diets, including the Atkins Diet, Weight Watchers, NutriSystem, and other diets the names of which she couldn't even remember. She told me she was fifty pounds overweight, and her self-loathing was obvious in nearly every sentence that came out of her mouth.

Using my program, combined with her already-acquired knowledge about herself, she recently reported that she has not dieted for over seven years and successfully maintains a healthy weight. Five years ago, Rebecca started her own physical therapy business. She now employs seven therapists and is very successful as a result of her savvy business sense and hard work. She finally realized that, like running her business, successfully maintaining a healthy weight could not be accomplished through some quick-fix gimmick.

Kathryn, another patient, sat in my office in tears, convinced that she would never lose the forty pounds she had regained *after* her stomach staple surgery three years earlier. She opted for the surgery after years of yo-yo dieting. She had been divorced for six years and saw herself growing old by herself "because no one would want [her]."

Kathryn is now working as a legal assistant on the East Coast. She feels much better about herself because she no longer uses self-negating statements to try to motivate herself. At our last communication, she reported that she continued to think differently about her body and how she cares for it. She has also lost forty pounds and assured me that she would never regain it.

These are two familiar scenarios, typical of how the diet culture can actually damage people. In most cases, my system can undo the damage. The human body is remarkable in its ability to adapt and heal, so don't let the past discourage you. Did you know that diet programs have the highest rate of consumer dissatisfaction of any service industry? Estimates of relapse rates among dieters range from 75 percent to 95 percent. One of the most comprehensive studies, carried out by Consumer Reports, indicates relapse rates are closer to 75 percent.

Understand this clearly: the weight loss strategy in this book is not about dieting. Because this strategy is not about dieting, I'm going to give you a list of guidelines for eating. (These are explained in detail in chapter 10.) Remember: DO NOT CALL THIS A DIET.

1. Limit your intake of refined sugar.
2. Limit your intake of refined carbohydrates.
3. Limit your intake of white flour.
4. Limit trans fat and fried foods.
5. Eat only *lean* red meat.
6. Increase your intake of fresh fruits and vegetables.
7. Reduce the size of the portions you serve yourself.
8. Always leave a little food on your plate when finished eating.

You need to understand why diets don't work, and in this chapter you will get the information you need to understand this. It will also help you to understand that lifestyle change—along with changes you make in your brain and the way you think about losing weight—is the way to lose weight consistently and permanently.

To date, I have never had anyone enter my weight loss program that had never been on a diet. In most cases, they came to me after having failed on several diets, taken various diet pills, and, in a few cases, had stomach staples.

Take a moment to consider the gastric bypass procedure, commonly known as stomach stapling. In 2003 alone, the American Society for Bariatric Surgery estimates that 103,200 people have had this surgery. By comparison, in 1998, there were only 25,800 obesity-related operations (mostly gastric bypasses). That is an increase of 400 percent, exactly what the bariatric equipment industry has forecast for growth in their market and sales potential. These industry marketing experts don't seem worried about losing sales, despite the millions of diet books out there on the shelves. They know they don't work. The scary part of these surgeries is the risk. You can find evidence of this in Associated Press (AP) articles over the wire to all the newspapers in the country, as two patients died from the surgery in New England.

Risks include wound infections, stomach leaks, and life-threatening blood clots. The International Bariatric Surgery Registry estimates that one of every one thousand patients who undergo the surgery will die within four weeks, and three in one thousand will die within three months. Some experts put the fatality number at one in a hundred!

According to the Associated Press, Ken Powers from Boston knew the risks but underwent the surgery anyway. At 475 pounds, he believed that it was worth taking the risk of dying on the operating table if the surgery could give him a better life than the way he was living. By the tens of thousands, morbidly obese (bariatric) people who have failed at diets, support groups, and exercise programs are turning to surgery as a last resort. Insurance carriers have started to pay for the procedure, calculating that it's cheaper than treating the health-related problems associated with obesity, such as diabetes and high blood pressure.

Powers is now concerned about how weatherman Al Roker and singer Carnie Wilson make it look simple and convenient, especially for young people. He says that you don't see all of the post-surgical pain and complications involved, like throwing up after eating only half an English muffin. It takes a year, he says, to be able to eat certain foods again.

There is plenty of evidence that stomach staple surgery is a bad choice, and a very risky one at that. Surgery, diet pills, and gimmick diets are all attempts at quick fixes. It's obvious that dieting hasn't worked for these people, either. The program in this book is a strategy that works without risk.

One of the main reasons diet pills don't work is that the function of the pill is to suppress the hunger response. Eating when you are hungry is not the problem; the problem is eating when you are not hungry. People become overweight because they eat when they are not hungry so suppressing the feeling of hungry does not help most who struggle with weight.

With my patients, it's obvious too. They've all tried dieting. If those diets (or even stomach staples) had worked for them, they would not have found their way to my office.

The word "diet" is defined as "food and drink regularly provided or consumed." "Diet" simply refers to our regular eating and drinking habits. Unfortunately, the word has been co-opted by our society and an entire industry to identify any one of a number of specialized food regimens. The "diets" usually connote a short-term regimen that one "goes on" and follows until a desired amount of weight has been lost.

While these diets do offer some good suggestions to help you lose weight, they also offer unrealistic expectations, are often too narrow in their focus, and usually offer very little to help motivate you to adhere to their program. Their proponents tout high protein, low carbohydrate, too much fat, too little fat, counting calories, and counting fat grams, none of which really help you take off weight for the long term. They are often too exclusionary of certain foods and too specific about what you should eat, which makes adherence to them difficult. If reading a diet book worked to help you lose weight, you would have lost excess weight a long time ago. There are millions of books in print touting it. There are new diet books on the stands every month, as they are the new fad in publishing. DIET BOOKS DO NOT HELP YOU LOSE WEIGHT PERMANENTLY.

Choosing good food is part of the picture, though, and this book incorporates what I think is the best of what Atkins (*New Diet Revolution*), Ornish (*Eat More, Weigh Less*), and Sears (*The Zone*) have to offer in that regard, but I do not call it a diet. It is only one aspect of the lifestyle changes that can occur by changing your brain. Remember, you are not changing your brain to go on another diet. You are changing your brain to launch a new lifestyle.

I agree that the body needs a lot of protein, as the Atkins diet recommends. That's a sound idea. However, I completely disagree with the sources he suggests. Don't ignore the accompanying danger when you consume excessive, inferior, and unhealthy sources of protein such as red meat, bacon, sausage, and certain cheeses. Proponents of the Atkins diet are now recommending less red meat in the diet. These changes make this diet confusing and difficult to follow for very long. You can eat combinations of vegetables, whole grains, nuts and seeds, low-fat dairy, protein shakes, chicken, fish, and reduced quantities of lean red meat for the protein you need. If you buy red meat, buy the leanest meat available.

In my opinion, the Atkins diet's charge that carbohydrates are the culprit in weight gain is simply preposterous. You will gain weight only if you eat the wrong kinds of—and too many—carbohydrates.

The *Eat More, Weigh Less* diet also provides a few sound ideas for weight loss, but the drastic reduction in fat intake is extremely hard on your body, especially your skin. You may lose some weight temporarily on this diet, but you can also lose the vitality of your skin. Remember, there are good and poor sources of fat, just as with protein.

The Zone Diet recommends 30 percent fat, which I believe to be excessive.

Although I make recommendations about the balance of carbohydrates, proteins, and fats, I don't believe that a strict adherence is imperative if you are getting nutrients from appropriately healthy sources. Thirty percent fat, as *The Zone Diet* suggests, is just too much. Ideally, your balance of carbohydrates, protein, and fat should be 40 to 45 percent, 35 to 40 percent, and 15 to 20 percent, respectively.

Many of these diets require special foods and rules, thus taking away the individual's need to develop better eating habits and become a responsible decision maker. These diets are difficult to follow in social situations, not to mention in daily life in general. It is questionable whether any of these diets work long-term for anyone, no matter if they are specialized diets such as NutriSystem, Weight Watchers, Atkins, or Sugar Busters, or those claiming a twenty-four-hour turnaround, a method of outwitting your weight, the promise of a fat flush plan, a five-day miracle diet, or the suggestion that you can eat, cheat, and melt away the fat. The specialized diets can be expensive and the pie-in-the-sky promises are, more often than not, ridiculous.

In nutritional and psychological literature there is considerable research and a general consensus that diets do not work. Long-term studies on thousands of people show that "dieting is a notoriously ineffective means of achieving weight loss."

One of the reasons diets don't work is because they involve a cookie-cutter mentality. By this, I mean that there is an assumption that anyone can lose weight on a particular diet. However, because we are not all created equal, what works for one person may not work for the next.

Diets also don't work because of the unrealistic expectations held by both men and women. Women generally expect to lose between two and three pounds per week, and men expect to lose between three and four pounds. More often than not, when those expectations are not met, adherence to the diet stops.

The proponents of many of these diets would also have you believe that they are "based on a new nutritional principle that makes weight loss virtually automatic, thus requiring little if any effort on the part of the dieter." However, losing weight requires a new mindset. It requires work, perseverance, effort, and a belief in yourself. You can lose weight if it is important enough to you, and you have the tools in this book to lose it the right way.

There may be as many reasons why diets fail as there are dieters, and this is why my program involves lifestyle change and not dieting. My program involves a dramatic change in the way you think about losing weight, and the resulting lifestyle changes are tailored for you—by you. With the exception of suggestions of certain foods to limit, my patients basically create their own regimen. Research has shown that the success rate is actually higher for people who manage their own weight loss program than for those who seek the assistance of formal programs.

Proponents of the diets do not realize the psychologically harmful effects that unrealistic expectations can cause: "feelings of frustration and defeat, guilt, self-hatred, and depression."

How does an industry that fails so miserably continue to thrive so tremendously, bringing in as much as $40 billion annually? Janet Polivy and Peter Herman suggest in *American Psychologist* that there are probably two reasons for this: big promises and repeat customers. The promises attract people and the magnitude of the promises practically guarantees failure. For reasons not clearly understood, these repeated failures do not seem to deter people from trying yet another diet. The mere act of purchasing another diet book or making the decision to try another diet has an immediate, positive effect. This effect is probably very similar to the measurable improvement in distressed individuals after simply making a telephone call to schedule an appointment with a psychotherapist.

The good news is that anyone who eventually loses weight and keeps it off has almost always failed on previous attempts, just as with quitting smoking. It is time for you to see your past failures as the catalyst that got you where you are now. You've taken the failure route; you've paid your dues. This is your time for success. Believe it!

Believe it because you are not going on another diet; instead, you are going to see losing weight in a new context as a result of reading this book. I am not making pie-in-the-sky promises; rather, I will motivate you to do what it takes to lose weight the right way. You will lose weight by finally taking responsibility for yourself and your daily decisions. You will be able to change your brain circuitry, reducing your cravings to overeat, and reducing your cravings to eat the wrong kinds of food. You will find a renewed energy that you have never had in the past because you will see your effort as something you are capable of sustaining. Your thought processes will be dramatically different as a result of reading this book and following my program.

You must understand that I have also followed the compulsive dieting route. It was not fun, and I was not successful. I have learned, however, what it takes to stay at a healthy weight without dieting. I practice what I preach.

When I was a compulsive dieter in the seventies, a number of strange diets abounded. I remember going on a grapefruit diet, a hard-boiled egg diet, and a cabbage-and-buttermilk diet (the most unusual). Every day for lunch I had a cup of cabbage and a half cup of buttermilk. Someone's dad was on it and had lost twenty pounds, so why not give it a try?

After trying several of these diets, I became extremely frustrated and developed an unhealthy disease known as anorexia nervosa. I was convinced that the only way I could ever control my weight was to starve myself. I remember going days at a time eating next to nothing. On a five-foot, six-inch frame, I got down to around ninety pounds. I had an extreme body image distortion, as I continued to feel fat at that weight. My hair began to fall out, my complexion deteriorated, I stopped menstruating, and I couldn't grow fingernails. Because I had no body fat, I was so cold in the winter that I could hardly stand to go outside.

Somehow, without professional help, I got control over my problem. I was luckier than most anorexics. Many spend years in psychotherapy, and some eventually die from it.

Luckily, my only attempt at purging after bingeing was unsuccessful; otherwise, I might have become bulimic. It is difficult to talk about those experiences; however, I want you to know that you can learn healthy weight control and overcome your difficulty with food.

I also remember when I finally began to exercise and went on a high-protein diet. I do not ever remember feeling so consistently miserable. My main exercise was running and I continued to wonder when I was going to experience a runner's high. Since I was consuming no carbohydrates, I had no energy. I was basically running on empty. I would come in from a four-mile run and eat cottage cheese, turkey, and a hard-boiled egg. It truly astounds me that there are still diet gurus out there touting strict, high-protein diets. I will never be convinced that bananas and carrots are bad for me.

There is a lot of controversy surrounding the high-protein diets such as Sugar Busters and Atkins. Critics suggest that the meat and high-fat dairy products these diets permit cause artery-clogging saturated fats to accumulate in the blood vessels. Most of the weight that is lost is water weight as a result of the body processing proteins rather than carbohydrates for energy. You also limit your intake of grains, nuts, vegetables, and fruit, which provide dietary fiber, vitamins, minerals, and the anticancer phytochemicals that are found only in plant foods.

Another reason high-protein, low-carbohydrate diets are so dangerous is that your brain may not get the sugar (glucose) it requires to function. All organs in your body require food for energy. Organs other than your brain can use fats and proteins for energy; however, your brain requires a steady source of glucose for energy. Without this steady source, you can experience diminished mental performance as well as the energy depletion or "blah" feeling described above. There is some speculation about a connection between a long-term diminished supply of glucose to the brain and dementia and more concrete evidence suggesting a correlation between obesity and Alzheimer's.

The lethargic feeling from low blood sugar is extremely uncomfortable and—because the body can tolerate extremely low carbohydrate intake for only a limited time—most people don't last very long on these diets. Considering the health risks, it is probably a good thing that they don't.

It is unrealistic to think that you can drastically change your eating habits until you have lost the desired weight, and then expect to keep it off when you go back to your old—often unhealthy—eating habits. Many patients report that when their bodies can no longer tolerate the absence of carbohydrates in their diet, they still end up eating high-protein and high-fat foods, and then add carbohydrates due to uncontrollable urges for carbs. Thus, they are right back where they began. These diets are not about developing good decision-making techniques, but about giving up control to a specific set of rules. After all, your daily food consumption is a complex series of decisions and the sooner you learn to make responsible decisions, the sooner you can expect to lose weight consistently and permanently. Once you begin to experience the change in your brain circuitry, your decision making becomes much easier.

Understanding the physiology of dieting can help you understand why dieting does not work. When you begin to lower your caloric intake, your body gradually and automatically adjusts its metabolism to compensate for the decrease in calories. You see, at the cellular level, your body responds as if you are going into starvation mode. Once your intake goes below a certain level, your metabolism will almost shut down because it fears no more food is going to be consumed. This is why dieters so quickly reach a plateau and stop losing weight. The only ways to speed up your metabolism healthily are to exercise and build additional muscle mass.

It is unrealistic to believe you can lose weight simply by lowering your caloric intake. As Covert Bailey writes in *The New Fit or Fat*, "Any diet book that claims permanent weight loss without exercise is counterfeit."

Lowered caloric intake explains why people stranded on a deserted island can survive for such long periods of time, provided water is available. In such a situation, the body really does go into starvation mode, and it's possible to lose so much weight in the form of fat that one will then begin to lose muscle mass as well. Losing muscle further slows the metabolic rate since muscle mass works as a motor to speed up your metabolism.

You should also know that the process of losing significant weight and regaining it over and over again is extremely dangerous. There may be actual health risks from yo-yo dieting, such as lower HDL (good cholesterol), which is associated with an increased risk of heart attack. It has not been documented, but personal reports from many of my patients indicate that with each cycle, the weight, plus as much as an additional 10 percent, often returns more quickly and the subsequent loss is more difficult.

For all the above reasons, I do not allow my patients to consider their adherence to my plan as dieting. We strictly talk about lifestyle changes and changing your brain. I want to be very clear that I am talking about lifestyle change and how to do it, and that rapid weight loss is not a part of this program.

Michael Fumento writes in *The Fat of the Land:* "choose a regimen that emphasizes not speed but permanency." He suggests that expectations of losing two pounds a week is too much for most people. You must begin to think about slow, consistent, and permanent weight loss.

I will encourage you to expect to lose one pound per week and work very hard to be satisfied with that. Most of you do not need to lose fifty pounds, but in one year that is how much you would lose if you lost one pound a week. Forget about trying to get down to your ideal weight in a few months. You know that it has never worked in the past, so don't expect it to work now.

Portion control is another lifestyle change you will learn about. In addition to the smaller portions that you initially put on your plate, leaving a small amount of food behind on your plate will also help control your portions. The "leave a little" philosophy of eating will sometimes get attention when dining with guests. "Aren't you going to finish that?" and "Are you going to waste it?" are common questions they may ask. Keep in mind, it's better to waste it than to "waist" it. You can't let social pressure dictate your eating habits. Some of this goes back to being a child and having parents force children to clean their plate.

I am asking you to consider lifestyle changes that you intend to adhere to for the rest of your life. Initially, these will not be dramatic changes. One of these changes is exercise. For someone who doesn't exercise regularly, beginning an exercise program will probably be the most dramatic change. In chapter 8 you will find information to provide you with increased motivation to exercise and a self-hypnosis script to make it easier. Remember, the guided meditations provided in the script will help in changing your brain, which will make your decision to exercise much easier.

I hope that what you have read in this chapter has convinced you that dieting is not the way to lose weight. There may be diets that work for some people some of the time, but I am convinced that the psychological pressure you put on yourself trying to adhere to a program that has not been proven to work will, in the long run, create more problems than it solves. It will not do anything to change the urges that come from your brain. To succeed with weight loss, you must change your entire belief system about dieting—and learn to listen to, and appreciate, your body. Learning what works for you may not be an overnight process, but the long-term benefits can be very rewarding, especially as you begin changing the way you respond to old messages by using your will and positive self-talk to change your brain.

Self-hypnosis Script Three:
Decision Making

This segment is designed to enhance your decision-making power in various situations. As with most of the self-hypnosis scripts, this helps you to visualize yourself feeling confident and having the strength to make the right food choices. There is no question that the more you visualize yourself being successful, the more likely you are to be successful in real life situations. The premise here is that you are encouraged by what you visualize and your mind will begin to help you to block the unhealthy desires and change your brain. The more you repeat the script, the more it is internalized and becomes your own, and the more it affects your brain circuitry.

Find a comfortable lying or seated position.

Take two or three nice, deep breaths and begin to allow your body to relax. Keep your attention on your breathing for several seconds. Allow your belly to soften, and notice the breath as it passes in and out of your nostrils.

Let yourself be aware of the sensations within your body, the moment-to-moment sensations that occur with each inhalation and exhalation.

Notice how your body is beginning to relax into the cushions beneath you.

You will begin to feel heaviness in your body as you soften and loosen the muscles throughout your body.

As you begin to find yourself in a very pleasant state of relaxation, begin to see yourself in some of the situations in which you will find yourself over the next few days that will require you to make choices about the food you will put in your mouth.

See yourself at home, at work, out at your favorite restaurant, or visiting family and friends.

Also see yourself at various times of the day—at breakfast, lunch, and dinner.

See yourself making healthy food choices.

Get a very clear picture of yourself looking vibrantly healthy, wearing something you haven't been able to wear because of your weight gain.

That's right, you see yourself looking closer and closer to your ideal weight.

As you begin to visualize yourself in all of those situations, notice that your head is held a little higher and your shoulders are thrown back.

You are carrying yourself in a more confident manner because you know that you will not allow yourself to overeat or to eat the foods that are clearly no longer in your healthy lifestyle.

You also have a glimmer of hope and excitement in your eyes, and you are feeling very good about yourself.

You are feeling very confident that whatever food choices confront you, you are going to be able to make the correct ones.

Whether it is your friends, your mother, or anyone else who encourages you to eat something that is no longer in your lifestyle, you are feeling confident that you will maintain control and make the best choices for yourself.

That's right, you see yourself beginning to regain control of what goes into your mouth because you know that there are very few things in your life over which you have more control than what goes into your mouth.

With this image of yourself in your mind, take two or three deep, full breaths.

As you inhale, feel the confidence well up in your chest.

With your next deep breath, notice the psychological strength coursing through your veins.

Take one more deep breath, and notice the excitement in your body as you begin to feel centered in your resolve to make the right food choices for yourself in each of those situations.

You very much like seeing yourself wearing the clothing you've been unable to wear because of your weight gain.

It feels so good to you.

You know that, as you begin to internalize and grasp your newfound belief in your ability to control what you put in your mouth, you will also begin to see yourself as vibrantly healthy.

You are vibrantly healthy, radiantly beautiful, and fully in control of the decisions you will make.

No matter what situation you find yourself in, no matter the circumstances, you will not allow yourself to indulge in those old-fashioned, unhealthy eating habits at the risk of embarrassing yourself in front of your family, friends, and colleagues.

From now on, in a very interesting way, you will make the choices that are becoming second nature to you confidently and comfortably.

You are going to be in control and confident of the choices you make regarding the food you eat.

You are going to grasp the notion that "you are what you eat." That's right, you are what you eat, and you are going to protect what you are becoming.

You are going to increase your awareness of what you are eating, and you will notice that this greater awareness increases your ability to do something about it.

More and more, you will begin to enjoy the tastes of healthy foods and be aware of the process whereby the food becomes your body.

In a very interesting way, you will find that the idea that "you are what you eat" will give you increased motivation to eat healthily and to avoid poisonous foods.

That's right, you will avoid too much white flour, refined sugar, and fried foods.

Your newfound confidence is going to make avoiding those foods much easier than ever before.

You will not eat as much food, and the variety may not be as extensive, but you will begin to be completely satisfied with what you do eat.

You will be completely satisfied because you will pay attention to the aroma, appearance, taste, texture, and temperature of your food.

Not because I am telling you, but because of the power of your will to change your brain, you will be able to block the desire to overeat.

In a very interesting way, you are going to begin to block the discomfort of craving foods that are no longer in your lifestyle. Each healthy decision will strengthen the neural pathways in your brain to make the next decision easier.

Be proud, be very proud that you made the adult decision to protect your health and be clear in your mind that there is absolutely no need to overeat.

You are a very strong, very capable, and very caring adult, and you are now going to extend that care to yourself.

You will begin to feel a justifiable sense of pride for having worked toward and achieved such an important, healthy, and worthwhile goal.

Once again, take two or three deep breaths and just feel the psychological strength welling up in your chest.

Take another deep breath, and feel the confidence coursing through your veins.

That's right, you are feeling so good about yourself.

With your next deep breath, feel the excitement as you become very strong and centered in your resolve to maintain your lifestyle changes.

You feel that strength from the top of your head to the tip of your toes.

Just spend several seconds noticing how calm and relaxed you are feeling.

Notice that you are truly beginning to believe that no matter what the situation, regardless of the circumstances, you will maintain your lifestyle changes with a very minimal desire to overeat.

In a very interesting way, the visualizations and the messages you have given yourself are going to help you to cope completely with any desire to overeat.

With any desire to overeat you will relax, much like you are relaxed right now, and take a few deep breaths, allowing the confidence and psychological strength to help you to cope completely with any desires.

You will find that, each day, it will become easier and easier for you to make the healthy decisions to protect your body.

With this strategy, it will begin to feel very natural for you to treat yourself in a healthy, proper manner.

This strategy is strengthening your will, your will is strengthening your mind, and your mind is going to change your brain.

Your will can strengthen the neural pathways in your brain and weaken urges to overeat.

You are no longer an overeater. You are feeling a growing power within you to make healthy food choices and permanently lose weight.

Chapter Four

Why Do You Want to Lose Weight?

"Health…is the first and greatest blessing of all."
—Lord Chesterfield

One of the first questions I ask my patients is: "Why do you want to lose weight?" The answer gives me a lot of information about them, as well as their chances of adhering to their weight loss program. If someone comes in because a parent, spouse, or friend told them they needed to lose weight, I usually suggest they not waste their time and money. Consistent and permanent weight loss will occur only if you are doing it for yourself.

Most people who seek help for weight loss are long past adolescence and may have suffered from the debilitating effects of a mother who badgered them about their weight. Often, however, their mother has been replaced by a different person who is also inappropriately involved in their life. You will lose weight because *you* want to, not because they want you to.

Understand that your reasons for wanting to lose weight are very important. It is imperative that you consider your reasons very carefully and make sure that you have only your best interests in mind. As you read this chapter, try to get a better understanding of yourself and your real reasons for wanting to lose weight.

Probably the most frequent response to this question is appearance. Appearance is a viable reason for wanting to lose weight. Discrimination against overweight people has been regularly documented. Our society puts an extremely high premium on thinness, to the detriment of many young girls who have tried to attain an impossible standard that is paraded in front of them through all media outlets. Christiane Northrup, author of *Women's Bodies, Women's Wisdom*, believes that "almost all women in the United States have a body image distortion because of the millions of images of perfect airbrushed women that the media flash at us constantly." These images create a tendency to relate to one's body through negative comparisons. *People* magazine describes the result: "Society's standard of beauty is an image that is literally just short of starvation for most women."

It is of paramount importance for you to start where you are right now and accept who you are. Of course, you bought this book because you would like to lose weight, but until you accept where you are right now, losing weight will be very difficult. I am not asking you to be happy with your weight; I am asking you to be accepting of yourself in your entirety. Your body is a very important component of who you are, but you know that you have much more to offer than a body. If you are relying on your physical appearance to make you who you are and to gain acceptance from others, you are barking up the wrong tree. Your value as a person must come from your own assessment, not from those around you.

Take an inventory of the many wonderful things you have to offer to others in your life. Every day of your life, you give of yourself in many ways. You give your time, attention, and care to those around you. If you can begin to value yourself more for the many good qualities you possess, you will find that your obsession with your physical appearance will become less important. Paradoxically, as your obsession decreases, your appearance will probably improve.

Of course, caring about how you look is a strong indicator of how much you value yourself and what is important to you. It reveals to the outside world that you care about yourself and your health. Just make sure that you are realistic about your expectations. Next time you pick up a fashion magazine, remember that these models have been airbrushed to perfection and represent a minority. Avoid the comparison game. You have much more to offer than just looking pretty in front of a camera.

Good health is the second most frequent response to why people want to lose weight. It seems that this ought to be the other way around; however, given our society's obsession with appearance, it is not surprising. *Psychology Today* reported that 41 percent of survey respondents would give up five years of their life in order to be thin. How about being thin and keeping those five years?

While appearance may be the most important reason for my patients to lose weight, it may be their overemphasis and possible obsession with appearance that has made losing weight so difficult. While we're the fattest industrialized nation in the world, we're also the most obsessed with thinness. There has to be a connection between the overweight epidemic in the United States and this obsession.

It is my belief that, if a shift in focus occurs here, there is a better chance for my patients to lose weight. At the juncture in most of my patients' lives when they come to me, the most important goal in life ought to be their health. As we will see in chapter 5, obesity is responsible for a whole host of health problems. If you don't have your health, little else in life matters.

However, a person's appearance can be the complete opposite of what is going on inside. A common weight-loss strategy, unfortunately, is bingeing and purging (commonly known as bulimia), and though bulimics may appear healthy on the outside, a very different picture unfolds on the inside.

I try to instill the mindset in my patients that, yes, they want to lose weight, but they are really here for their health. Your goal should be to die young as late in life as possible. Do you like the idea of lengthening the time and quality of life with those who are important to you?

Life insurance companies know about dying young as late in life as possible. I have had two patients recently who cited lower rates for their life insurance policies as a reason for wanting to lose weight. Jim, who has lost seventy pounds in the last ten months, told me he will save nearly five thousand dollars per year in personal and business life insurance costs because of his weight loss.

Vicky came into my office a few years ago after the birth of her first grandchild. She said she had no idea that she would get this kind of pleasure from a grandchild. This may not have been her only motivation for wanting to lose weight, but it was certainly important to her to be able—over the next several years—to see this child grow up, graduate from college, marry, and share many more wonderful experiences with him.

She made some lifestyle changes, and chasing after her now three-year-old grandson is not her main form of exercise. She goes to the gym four or five days a week and cares for him three days a week. Vicky reports that her new attitudes about eating greatly influence what she eats and what she feeds her grandson as well.

The desire to feel better physically motivates a lot of people to lose weight. The simple act of carrying around extra weight creates a great deal of discomfort. I watch obese people actually struggle to get in and out of the chairs in my office. Getting in and out of a car can be a major task. Even putting on shoes is difficult. Obesity restricts individual freedom to engage in even the simplest of social activities.

Self-esteem is another commonly cited reason for wanting to lose weight. In fact, one of my patients said, "I feel like I have more confidence when I am thinner." There is no question that self-esteem and appearance are related, but failure to control your eating is as much a cause of poor self-perception as your appearance. Every time you are confronted with a food choice, you have an opportunity to raise your self-esteem. The more often you opt for the correct food choice, the quicker you tip the self-esteem scale in a positive direction.

Wanting to feel more in control of one's life is a very good reason for wanting to lose weight. Can you think of anything in your life over which you have more control than what goes into your mouth? Probably not. We live in a permeable society in which we impinge upon, and are impinged upon, constantly. As much as we would like to consider ourselves free and independent, it is simply not the case. Paying taxes, getting along with others close to us, enduring the weather, and dying are just a few of the things over which we have only varying degrees of control. Most of us like to be in control, and it appears that we often work harder at trying to control the uncontrollable things in our lives than we do at controlling the food choices that are constantly in front of us. When you give up your efforts to control inappropriately, you will find that you have a reservoir of strength to control what goes into your mouth. An interesting side note is that once people begin to control their eating, their level of control improves over a whole host of other controllable things, such as money spending and temper.

So why have so many people relinquished control over what they eat? In addition, why are we constantly intellectualizing about the loss of control? Frequently, I will have a patient lamenting, "Why do I crave and eat that? Why don't I adhere to my admonishments? What happened in my childhood that causes me to overeat?" I have to remind them continually that the answers to these questions, however intriguing, will not stop them from overeating. My advice to them is to stop intellectualizing over the past, get into their bodies, and get their thoughts into their new lifestyle—now! That is where we get results. When you finally start paying attention to what your body is saying to you and put it into the context of your new lifestyle, you will start changing your habits. Think about what your body feels like the next morning after gorging on a box of cookies and a bag of popcorn—as opposed to a halibut steak, salad, and broccoli.

I also have many patients who want to set a short-term goal of losing weight for some significant event. Julia came in for weight loss counseling because she was going to her twenty-five-year class reunion in a few months. It is completely unrealistic to think you can lose a significant amount of weight healthily in such a short period of time. I highly recommend against this because, so often, once the event has passed, the weight is regained. We are also seeing that the gain often exceeds the weight that was originally lost.

Julia did lose eight pounds before her reunion. It was certainly not as much as she had hoped to lose, but for several months thereafter she consistently lost just under one pound per week. She is now holding steady at about thirty-five pounds less than when she initially came in.

It is extremely important to consider your weight loss as a long-term endeavor. When I talk about lifestyle change—and I will talk about it frequently—I am referring to changing the rest of your life.

Your reasons for losing weight are going to influence whether you will lose weight and keep it off. All of the reasons mentioned—appearance, health, extended time with loved ones, self-esteem, and greater feelings of control—are potential contributors to enhanced quality of life. I want you to begin thinking about your current quality of life and what is really important to you. If you have your priorities in the right place, there is a really good chance that you will finally be able to take off those extra pounds—once and for all.

Self-hypnosis Script Four:
Die Young as Late in Life as Possible

There are many reasons to lose weight, and, in this chapter, we reviewed many of them. As noted, all of them involve your quality of life. In this segment, you will begin to incorporate a desire to lose weight for just that reason—to enjoy a youthful, healthy body as long as possible.

In a very comfortable setting, begin to take some nice, deep breaths.

With each inhalation, feel your chest expanding, and with each exhalation, imagine the tightness and tension dissipating out of your body.

With each exhalation, begin to clear your mind of all the thoughts of your day.

Each time you exhale, you allow yourself to become a little more relaxed.

You begin to feel your body sinking into the cushions beneath you, becoming more and more calm and relaxed with each exhalation.

You will find that the more relaxed you become, the more receptive you will be to your own thoughts.

The messages that you will read will become more acceptable to you, and you will find yourself believing that losing weight will become very important to you so that you might enjoy a higher quality of life.

Losing weight and protecting your health will become your highest priority.

You know that, at this time in your life, your health is the most important goal to pursue.

Your body is the precious physical entity through which you experience your life. If you want to experience your life to its fullest, you must respect and protect your body.

Your body is the home of your spirit.

Begin to create a picture of yourself in your mind looking and feeling optimally healthy.

Picture yourself at your ideal weight and notice how good that feels to you.

You may want to see yourself engaging in an activity you performed in the past, but are no longer able to do because of your weight.

Begin to notice how pleasing that image is to you.

See yourself wearing something you no longer wear because of your weight gain.

Notice how much you like that image.

Notice how vibrantly healthy you look.

Because you want to experience and enjoy your life to the very fullest—and you know that it is very important to you—you will begin to protect your body.

It will begin to feel very natural to protect and respect your body.

You will begin to protect every cell, every fiber, and every organ within your body.

It is true that overeating or consuming unhealthy foods is not good for you and you are against this, but your emphasis will now be upon your commitment to work toward a healthy body.

Because of this emphasis, it is going to feel natural for you to protect your body against the poison and pollution of overeating.

That's right—you will begin changing your lifestyle and it will feel very natural to you.

You can see yourself looking vibrantly healthy and radiantly beautiful.

You will begin to treat your body as though it is very fragile and precious.

Every moment of your life occurs through your body.

Every thought, every feeling, and every experience occurs through your body.

You are excited about your thoughts, feelings, and experiences occurring through your healthy body.

You know that your appearance is important to you, but as you begin to emphasize your health, your obsession with your appearance becomes less important and it becomes easier to lose weight.

That's right—your obsession with appearance diminishes as your emphasis on health increases.

You will begin to see yourself as your body's keeper in a very interesting way. You are, in truth, your body's keeper.

You know that your self-esteem is based upon, among other things, behavior that makes you feel good about yourself, and eating healthily will boost your self-esteem.

Eating healthily will make you feel better and better about yourself.

You will not allow yourself to indulge in overeating behavior that, in effect, will lower your self-esteem.

Each healthy choice will strengthen your self-esteem and diminish negative self-talk.

Every time you make the healthy choice, you are enhancing the quality of your life and making the next healthy choice easier.

You are continuing to see yourself making healthy choices and it feels very good to you. As you see yourself making healthy choices, take a nice, deep breath and feel the confidence coursing through your veins. Feel the psychological strength welling up in your chest.

Be assured that your mind is changing your brain. The urges to make unhealthy choices are diminishing and healthy choices are becoming easier.

Losing weight requires an almost constant series of choices throughout your day, and you will find those healthy choices becoming easier and easier.

Be very clear in your mind that you can make the choice that will lead to a longer, healthier life.

You will be thrilled and delighted by how much easier the healthy choices will become.

That's right—each and every day you make a series of decisions that can and will enhance the quality of your life.

In a very interesting way, your quality of life will improve with each healthy decision that you make.

It will begin to get easier and easier to put the quality of your life before poor food choices.

You want to die young as late in life as possible.

Because of your desire to die young as late in life as possible, you will begin to live your life in a healthy and proper manner, and it will feel very natural to you.

Your body is the vehicle through which you enact your belief, and your belief in living your life in a healthy, proper manner is one of your most cherished beliefs.

You can—and you will—make more and more healthy choices each and every day.

Not because I am telling you and you are reading this, but because these words are becoming your own.

You are feeling these words in your heart center, and your attitudes are slowly, but surely, changing.

Your old identity as an overeater is being replaced by a new identity.

You now have the identity of a healthy eater.

You can actually see yourself in your mind's eye as a healthy eater, looking vibrantly healthy.

Remain totally relaxed and calm as you feel your new identity in your heart center.

Your new identity as a healthy eater will ensure that you die young as late in life as possible.

Chapter Five

Why Do You Overeat?

"Nothing is more debilitating than the dread associated with
immoderation in any area of our lives."
—Rolf Gates

Given all the good reasons to lose weight, why is 50 to
75 percent of the adult population in America
overweight? This is not a terribly productive question,
and it's certainly no excuse for being overweight. It becomes
especially unproductive if your reasons for overeating make it
easier for you to do so. Labeling someone with a diagnosis or
disease simply makes it easier for them to make excuses—and
less likely to take responsibility for their problem. As a good
friend of mine says about almost any situation, "If you need an
excuse, any excuse will do."

In my private practice, I work out of what I refer to as a
health model, as opposed to a *disease model*. This flies in the face

of how psychologists are forced to practice now. In order to receive third-party insurance payment, a diagnosis must be given. Obviously, you need to know what the problem is in order to treat it, but I believe too much emphasis is placed on disease. Overeating is not a disease. However, in this differentiation, I do exclude treating eating disorders—such as bulimia and anorexia nervosa—from my weight loss program because they are problems that need to be addressed differently.

In the eighteen years since I began developing this program, I have probably heard every imaginable reason for overeating. Some of those reasons have been unique, and my patients were sometimes convinced that they had legitimate reasons for overeating. However, there are no good reasons for overeating—only poor excuses.

A lot is written today about food addiction. There is only inconclusive evidence such a thing as food addiction even exists—and is it truly an addiction? There may be bodily reactions to a certain food that increase the likelihood to want more of that particular food, but to label this as an addiction seems counterproductive. It seems more of an obsession or a compulsion than it does an addiction.

There is plenty of research indicating that our bodies metabolize simple sugars quickly, which, in turn, raises blood-sugar levels. This energy surge occurs quite rapidly and counteracts lethargy. There is no question that this bodily response might cause a craving for sugar and create the potential to eat too much of it. Still, I don't think that referring to sugar consumption as an addiction is productive. This thinking can provide an excuse to eat too much sugar too often, with a belief that the necessary control from within cannot overcome the "addiction." This simply is not true. It can be overcome.

Moreover, I have had many patients report what they believe to be a carbohydrate addiction. There are entire books written about this. Again, certain bodily reactions occur after eating large quantities of carbohydrates, but is it productive to call it an addiction?

If you have these problems with sugar or carbohydrates, it seems far more likely that you have simply become a compulsive eater of those foods. A compulsion is evidenced by repeated intense urges. You may have these urges, but I do not consider compulsive eating a disease and I certainly don't see it as a justification for overeating. We've talked about urges, how they originate, how to change your thinking, how to rewire your brain, how to get control over them, and how to get them to diminish (and even go away completely). This is what you need to focus your thoughts on, not disease or addiction. You are not helpless. Your will can overcome these urges. Remember this. It will serve you well in your pursuit of a new lifestyle.

The act of eating, in and of itself, is highly overrated. Food is here to nurture our bodies, period. That is not to say that there is anything wrong with enjoying a good meal. I highly recommend it on a regular basis. However, many people overeat simply because there is so much emphasis on eating in our society. There is a lot of pressure to eat more often than you ought to and to eat more than you need. Restaurants are notorious for serving large portions. Overeating commonly occurs at restaurants because of large portion sizes, and because of the seductive hype of commercials. Think about how you feel after overeating. You are letting society and the media shove this stuff down your throat. Don't buy it. It's overrated and not good for you.

Fast-food restaurants, movie theaters, and convenience stores are now offering everything—in super size!—at incredible bargains. How can you pass it up? So what if a regular Coke and large fries is already more than you need? You can super size for only fifty cents more! This is a ploy to appeal to your sense of greed and the idea that you are getting something for next to nothing. It's an appeal to your mercantile sense of a great bargain. Are you tricked into believing that this is a good value? Are you going to be tricked into super sizing your body? When you read what's in this book later about trans fat, I'm hoping you won't want any more French fries—ever.

What about the plague of free food? This can include anything from free samples at the grocery store to the second and third helpings at a buffet restaurant. Just because food is there and it is free doesn't mean you have to eat it.

In our office, pharmaceutical representatives often bring us snacks. At least nine out of ten times the food they bring is unhealthy, like donuts, cookies, or candy. Donuts and cookies are generally loaded with trans fat. And to think that these representatives are in the health industry! What would be wrong with less of the aforementioned "treats" and more fruit and vegetable trays?

As a child, were you ever rewarded with food? Cynthia, a patient of mine, talks about how her mother gave her very little physical affection or praise when she was growing up. However, she often rewarded and comforted her with food. As an adult, Cynthia also learned to comfort herself with food when she was depressed, angry, or disappointed. Greater awareness of this habit helped her considerably. Cynthia also wrote a letter (it was never sent, but acted simply as a therapeutic assignment) to her mother. She was able to vent some anger and allow herself to acknowledge and cope with the sadness she experienced as a result of her mother's lack of affection. By letting go of some of her anger toward her mother, she experienced much less need for food to comfort her or to numb herself to her feelings. Is there someone in your life to whom a letter might alleviate some "stuffed" feelings?

I remember going to the doctor's office as a child and being given a sucker after getting a shot. Teachers often use food for rewards, too. When you think about it, it's really not that surprising that we grow up seeing food as something other than a way to nurture our bodies. You probably deserve to be rewarded on a regular basis, but there are better ways to do it than with food.

Consider this: thin and overweight people have distinctly different attitudes about themselves, their eating habits, and their bodies. The first major difference between thin attitudes and fat attitudes is the notion that you eat to live, rather than live to eat. Someone who lives to eat spends a great deal of time thinking about food. Immediately upon awakening and as soon as one meal is over, they are thinking about what they'll eat next. This is obsessive. Many people are obsessed with food in this society and think about it all the time. Remember, a thin person *eats to live*. You can still enjoy food, but if you have the attitude that you are eating to live, you are likely to eat more responsibly and with less guilt.

A related—but slightly different—attitude involves seeing food as fuel. Eating is similar to filling up your gas tank at the gas station. If you reason like a thin person, you replace the nozzle when the tank is full. This is unlike a fat attitude, in which after your tank is full you reason that there is more fuel, so why not fill up the trunk and backseat, too?

I am reminded of a TV commercial that tells us that we are what we eat, and a girl eating cinnamon rolls stands up, walks away, and has two very large cinnamon rolls fastened to her buttocks. So, the next time you eat beyond fullness, just imagine the extra food going straight to your backside. Or, better yet, food left on your plate after you are full should go into the refrigerator as leftovers or into the garbage. How does the image of treating yourself as a garbage can settle with you? It is certainly not an image I would like to entertain. Stop eating when your body feels full.

Another attitude involves eating by the clock. When people with thin attitudes look at the clock at noon and are not hungry, they simply continue working, reasoning that if they get hungry in an hour or two, they can eat an apple or protein bar. They don't eat a whole meal when they are not hungry just because it is noon. People with fat attitudes reason that, if they don't eat right then, they will be starving by dinnertime. They are telling themselves that they have to eat. This is faulty logic. Our bodies do not function like clocks. For various reasons, we are not always hungry at the same time every day.

Weight control is about learning to listen to your body. It was interesting to me that, after I started paying very close attention to the sensations of hunger and fullness, my eating desires changed around my menstrual cycle. The day before and the day my period starts, I tend to be somewhat bloated and less hungry. The day after my period is over, I tend to be much hungrier. If I didn't pay attention to the fullness on those days before my period and ate by the clock, I have a feeling that it would be easy to put on a couple of extra pounds that month.

Many of my patients who have overeaten for years admit that they are very out of touch with the feelings of hunger and fullness. They have learned to ignore the sensation of fullness completely. People who grossly overeat may not have experienced hunger for so long that they have actually forgotten what it feels like. Evelyn Tribole and Elyse Resch in their book, *Intuitive Eating*, compiled a list of bodily sensations that occur when someone is hungry. These symptoms include: mild gurgling, gnawing or growling in your stomach, light-headedness, difficulty concentrating, uncomfortable stomach pain, irritability, faintness, and headache. You are probably also aware that food tastes much better when you are really hungry. However, it is important that you not let yourself go beyond pleasant hunger, since that will put you at risk of bingeing.

Janet, who started my program a couple of weeks ago, said that she is starting to appreciate slight, healthy tinges of hunger. There are three reasons to tolerate a little hunger. First of all, when you are hungry, it is a signal to you that your body is using up stored fats and sugars. Second, it is also a signal that you will be eating soon, and knowing you will eat soon feels good because we all enjoy eating. Third, food tastes so much better when you are hungry. As one of my patients said, "hunger is the best spice."

Another attitude involves dealing with outside pressure to overeat, whether it is from friends or partners in your life. It is a given that most social situations now involve eating. Parties are triggers for overeating. Unfortunately, even in other social settings there may be pressure to eat when you are not actually hungry. Think of going to visit your grandmother, who urges you to eat. She has nurtured you with food in the past and it is difficult for you to disappoint her. Cultural mores often suggest that a good host or hostess offer a guest something to eat or drink as a sign of welcome. A drink of water can suffice in this setting, as opposed to eating a whole plate of cheese and crackers and drinking a Coke. Usually, the guest can make the choice politely, without offending the host or hostess.

Amy, one of my patients, recently related a story of going out to lunch with her office staff. She had begun my weight loss program, and cheeseburgers and French fries were something she ate only rarely (which was an especially good thing when you consider the trans fat content of these items). She ordered a chef salad with only half the cheese. She said that she felt as if she was betraying her friends, who ordered their usual cheese-burgers and French fries, dripping with trans fat. She said that, at times, it felt as if her friends actually ridiculed her. Overall, however, she was happier with her choice and proud of making it. Another patient, Anne, said her friends blatantly urged her to order fast foods because they felt that she was going to get too skinny. This fat attitude demands that you consider others' needs rather than your own when you decide what to eat. Are they thinking about you when they do this? No. They want you to fit into their lifestyle, not your own. You don't have to eat junk food just to fit in.

Because I have followed this program for many years, I am slender. Very frequently, my peers will encourage or even pressure me to overeat, or to eat something that is no longer included in my lifestyle. Several years ago, when I first changed my lifestyle, it was sometimes difficult to say "no" to their insistence that I indulge with them in their bad habits. At the very least, I would be compelled to explain why I wasn't going to eat something. This dynamic probably came from an old habit of trying to please others or taking care of others' needs at the expense of my own when I was growing up. If you choose to offer an explanation, simply be courteous and try not to make it a lecture.

As you can see, your attitudes toward yourself and others can greatly influence your eating habits. You may need to take an inventory of your attitudes and see if you have been overeating as a result.

I have worked with numerous individuals who consume a lot of food out of rebelliousness or a power struggle with parents, spouses, or other significant people in their lives. A sixteen-year-old female named Morgan, whom I saw for weight control, talked at length about how her mother constantly badgered her about the amount of food she was eating. Her mother forced her on diets when she was young and occasionally ridiculed her for her size. Morgan said that she would eat certain foods around her mother just to prove her independence—or, even worse, to make her mother mad.

Morgan worked hard to understand her misguided reasons for eating. She became more assertive with her mother, telling her she was capable of monitoring her own eating habits. Morgan works part-time at a local coffee shop, makes above-average grades in school, and plans to go to college. She wonders why her mother thinks she has to be so involved in her eating.

Adolescence is a critical stage in the development of one's identity. If you are not allowed to make your own decisions (food decisions are simply one of many areas) or are often criticized for the ones you do make, it certainly hampers your identity development. Many youngsters become rebellious if their parents interfere too much at this stage. This is the time for parents to begin weaning themselves off of the job of parenting, and removing themselves from the equation of food choice is a good place to start.

Another woman I worked with recently came in for help after giving birth to her third child. She was having a great deal of difficulty losing weight. When discussing her roadblocks, she burst into tears and said her husband refused to make love to her until she lost at least fifteen pounds. How motivated would you be in response to that kind of an ultimatum? She was having considerable difficulty separating her anger at her husband from her desire to lose weight.

Eunice, another patient who had changed her lifestyle and was beginning to lose weight, was confronted with an opposite reaction from her husband. They had been married for many years and, for most of those years, Eunice had been overweight. When she started losing weight, her husband started bringing home her old favorite treats (ice cream sandwiches, candy bars, etc.). She told him continually that she no longer ate those things, but could not convince him to stop buying them. The more weight she lost, the grumpier he became.

It became apparent that he was threatened by her increasing attractiveness due to weight loss. He felt safe and secure in the relationship as long as Eunice was obese, but the fear of other men finding her attractive was extremely difficult for him. Several sessions of marriage counseling helped to convince him that she was losing weight for herself. If their relationship benefited from her weight loss, it would be an added bonus for the two of them.

Alice, a very attractive woman who teaches at a local junior college, said that she cannot believe how often her anger at her husband triggers eating. He is one of those overly-involved partners who badgers her about her weight. She has gained close to twenty pounds since they married eight years ago. Her statement to me was, "He doesn't deserve a Barbie wife." Alice is a truly beautiful woman, but the extra weight definitely detracts from her beauty and harms her health.

Some of these examples required some therapy beyond weight-loss counseling. They do, however, highlight how interpersonal conflict can lead unconsciously to overeating or resistance to losing weight. Greater awareness, in and of itself, can lead to improvement.

Over the years, I have had a number of women come in for weight-loss counseling who were raped or sexually abused when they were younger. A very unfortunate phenomenon often occurs in these cases: there is a fear of being attractive to men. Because thinness is equated with attractiveness, it is difficult for them to get down to their ideal weight for fear of getting into a relationship in which intimacy is expected. This may be subconscious, but it is certainly a reason why some people overeat.

Stimuli to develop bad habits are everywhere: on television, in newspapers and magazines, and on billboards. It is extremely important to learn to be aware of these stimuli and stop and think before you indulge. At a recent meeting of the World Health Organization, there was some discussion about the advertising of unhealthy foods aimed at children. Recently, there was a one-hour television program dedicated to this issue, which raised the question about legislation prohibiting it. The food industry is targeting children—who are too young to see through the gimmicks—to persuade them to pressure their parents to buy bad food for them. This contributes to obesity and health problems in children (which coexist now in frightening proportions) who are too young to know the effect that eating bad foods has on the body. Keep your eye out for tempting ads about bad foods so that you and your children can successfully avoid them.

Emotional eating is another common reason for overeating. In the *International Journal of Eating Disorders*, Richard Ganley summarized more than fifty scientific studies and concluded that obesity is often a result of emotional eating. Many of the examples in this chapter involve overeating for emotional reasons. The moods that most often precede overeating are anger, anxiety, depression, loneliness, and boredom. All of these are negative emotions. Food becomes almost like a drug to you, and when you experience these negative emotions, you eat in order to numb yourself to them. Your craving for food may well be an indication of your emotional needs for nurturance that are not being met. There are more healthy sources for emotional nurturance.

There is also a rather common phenomenon of overeating that occurs as a result of a positive mood. Researchers at the University of Kansas found that overeating commonly occurs while celebrating a special occasion. As R.E. Thayer suggests in his book *Calm Energy*, a special celebration gives us license to break our dietary prohibitions and to indulge. Holidays are the most notable special occasions in which people tend to overeat. There is nothing wrong with indulging a little more than normal on holidays, but it is important to plan ahead for these occasions and not abandon your lifestyle changes completely. When the holidays are over, you will have to make up for that overindulgence.

Has overeating become a habit? According to Webster's definition, a habit is a constant, often unconscious, inclination to perform some act. Do you ever overeat out of habit? When I think of overeating out of habit, it is usually done at particular times of the day or in certain circumstances. That is not to say that you cannot develop good eating habits. One of the few good weight loss books available is *Habits Not Diets* by James Ferguson. Of course, in this book, we're talking about changing your thoughts and using your will to rewire your brain, which, in turn, will enable you to change bad habits into the good habits you need in your new lifestyle. Remember, when the brain changes, the urges are likely to support the new behavior.

In another light, there are many examples of overeating because of people in our environment and the influences they exert in our lives. If refusing to eat something someone offers you hurts their feelings or bothers them in any way, you must realize that it is not your problem. One of my patients who is overweight believes that if you are overweight, people are skeptical when you say no to food. If you are overweight, you may experience a little more pressure, which, in turn, may require more assertiveness. It is extremely important to learn to separate yourself from their feelings. If they are angry or upset with you, do not allow yourself to be deterred by their feelings. Remain constant in your resolve, in your solid sense of self. No one can make you feel anything you do not choose to feel. You can learn to be polite about turning down an offer for food you don't want to eat. People may not understand or know what you know. Learning to be courteous in these situations can allow you to be proud of your decisions and your ability to perceive the situation for what it is, and handle it smoothly. In the long run, it will only strengthen your resolve and pride.

Learning to take ownership of your feelings is extremely important. I spend a lot of time working with people on learning to acknowledge, label, and react to their feelings. Another book could be written on this. It is truly amazing to watch people learning to respond differently because they are finally able to look at a feeling, own it, and say to themselves, "Eating does not have to be my response to this feeling."

As you have just seen, and probably already knew, people overeat for many reasons. If you can become more aware of some of your reasons for overeating, you may be able to use better judgment in the face of those circumstances.

Chapter Six

Overeating Is Dangerous

*"As I see it, every day you do one of two things: build health
or produce disease in yourself."*
—Adelle Davis

No book on weight loss would be complete without a
discussion of just how dangerous it is to be
overweight. I don't believe that you overeat because
you lack awareness, but I believe it never hurts to be reminded
of the extreme danger in which you put yourself when you do.

Slow-motion suicide might sound a little severe for some
overweight individuals, but for those who suffer from
diabetes, have suffered a heart attack, or have high blood
pressure, it may not be far off the mark. When you see that
eating trans fat contributes dramatically to these health
problems as well, we're talking about things that can kill you.
Slow-motion suicide sounds a bit morbid and I don't believe

that you consciously want to kill yourself, but that may be exactly what you are doing. If your parents died at a young age from obesity-related diseases, it might not be as slow-motion as you think.

Perhaps an analogy I use with my patients preparing to stop smoking will help you to look at the dangers a little differently. If you brought home a bag of dog food from the store that said, "Warning: the surgeon general has determined that this dog food may be hazardous to your dog's health," would you feed it to your dog? Of course, everyone replies vehemently that they would not. Well, there is plenty of proof that obesity is as dangerous as smoking, so I think you can generalize this to the food you eat. You would not put your dog's health in danger, so why put yourself in harm's way? I believe that it is sometimes easier to feel compassion for our dogs and other significant individuals in our lives than for ourselves. Perhaps this analogy will help you to get a little more in touch with love, acceptance, and compassion for your own body.

Your body, regardless of genetics, is quite resilient. For most of us, our bodies will sustain considerable abuse before the damage begins to take its toll. Even if damage has already occurred, given your level of commitment, it is likely that you can rehabilitate your body. Our bodies, if we are kind to them, serve us very well.

Four hundred thousand people die annually as a result of complications resulting from obesity. As a result, society incurs as much as $117 billion per year in weight-related health care expenses. Experts estimate that between half and three-fourths of all adults in America are overweight. That's anywhere from 100 to 150 million people. Approximately nine million children are overweight.

Are you one of these overweight Americans? Typically, our only measure of whether we are overweight is the number found on the bathroom scale. While that information is important, it doesn't tell you how much of your weight is from muscle or fat. Consulting weight charts released by life insurance companies can be helpful, but even they don't take into consideration individual characteristics such as age. These charts don't tell you whether or not you are carrying around too much body fat and that is what distinguishes you as normal, overweight, or even obese. These insurance charts are included, however, because of their universal popularity and for those for whom the body mass index (BMI) does not apply.

The most widely used and meaningful guideline for determining the danger level for your weight is the body mass index. BMI is the average relative weight for height in people older than twenty years of age. It is usually correlated with body fatness and degree of disease risks, or how heavy you are relative to your height. It is extremely important to pay attention to the column which indicates the degree of risk to your health in which your BMI puts you.

But, first you need to calculate your BMI, and that's done as follows: weight (in pounds) multiplied by 705, divided by height, multiplied by height (in inches). Thus, one whose height is five feet seven inches (sixty-seven inches) and weighs 140 pounds, would calculate BMI this way:

140 multiplied by 705 equals 98,700
67 multiplied by 67 equals 4489
98,700 divided by 4489 = 21.9

The following table by Sizer and Whitney explains the different BMI measurements and their classifications:

BMI	OBESITY CLASS	RISKS TO HEALTH
<18.5	Underweight	Lower BMI, lower risk
18.5–24.9	Normal	Very low risk
25.0–29.9	Overweight	Increased risk/high risk
30.0–34.9	Class I obesity	High risk/very high risk
35.0–39.9	Class II obesity	Very high risk
40.0 & up	Class III obesity	Extreme risk

You are probably more familiar with the height-for-weight tables distributed by the Metropolitan Life Insurance Company, which take into account your body frame, gender, and height. By looking at the following charts, you can compare yourself with a population average and determine what is considered your ideal weight range.

MEN (Pounds)

HEIGHT	SMALL FRAME	MEDIUM FRAME	LARGE FRAME
5´2″	128-134	131-141	138-150
5´3″	130-136	133-143	140-153
5´4″	132-138	135-145	142-156
5´5″	134-140	137-148	144-160
5´6″	136-142	139-151	146-164
5´7″	138-145	142-154	149-168
5´8″	140-148	145-157	152-172
5´9″	142-151	148-160	155-176
5´10″	144-154	151-163	158-180
5´11″	146-157	154-166	161-184
6´0″	149-160	157-170	164-188
6´1″	152-164	160-174	168-192
6´2″	155-168	164-178	172-197
6´3″	158-172	167-182	176-202
6´4″	162-176	171-187	181-207

WOMEN (Pounds)

HEIGHT	SMALL FRAME	MEDIUM FRAME	LARGE FRAME
4´10″	102-111	109-121	118-131
4´11″	103-113	111-123	120-134
5´0″	104-115	113-126	122-137
5´1″	106-118	115-129	125-140
5´2″	108-121	118-132	128-143

5'3"	111–124	121–135	131–147
5'4"	114–127	124–138	134–151
5'5"	117–130	127–141	137–155
5'6"	120–133	130–144	140–159
5'7"	123–136	133–147	143–163
5'8"	126–139	136–150	146–167
5'9"	129–142	139–153	149–170
5'10"	132–145	142–156	152–173
5'11"	135–148	145–159	155–176
6'0"	138–151	148–162	158–179

If you did the BMI calculations and consulted the height-for-weight chart, you know how far outside your ideal adult weight range you fall and how much at risk you are for disease.

So what are the greatest dangers obesity wreaks on overweight individuals?

Although the physical and psychological effects of obesity cannot be separated entirely, the physical dangers need to be considered seriously. Heart disease, hypertension, and diabetes are the diseases most commonly associated with obesity. Several types of cancer are also associated with being overweight—most notably colon cancer, breast cancer, cervical cancer, and endometrial cancer. There is considerable research indicating that joint problems, especially of the knees, have a far greater likelihood of occurring in overweight individuals. As Dr. James Early suggested in a National Public Radio interview, if you are a hundred pounds overweight, it is like trying to land a 747 jet with Piper Cub landing gear. It does not work very well. Lower back pain also occurs more frequently in those who are overweight because your spine was not designed to carry anything more than your ideal weight.

Second only to smoking-related illnesses, obesity kills approximately four hundred thousand people each year. It is devastating to know that, in most cases, these premature deaths are completely preventable.

Because I am a psychologist, I see the psychological toll obesity is taking on my patients. Obesity exposes one to unfair prejudice. Ian K. Smith in his book *The Take Control Diet: a Plan for Thinking People* suggests that such prejudice begins early in life with not being chosen for school teams during recess and extends to employment opportunities, college acceptance, job earnings, and marital opportunities. Given the extensive bias against overweight individuals, it is no wonder that they suffer higher degrees of depression, anxiety, loneliness, and stress. Many of my patients are very depressed about their weight. There are those who argue that obesity is a result of depression. Whether the depression or the obesity came first, the fact is that a pervasive feeling of sadness often dominates the lives of obese individuals. They report feelings of hopelessness, as well as difficulty with motivation, concentration, and sleeping.

Anxiety concerning constant food choices can be extremely distressing. Anxiety, which can lead to even more health problems, is often high because of the fears associated with the potential physical dangers of obesity.

I have seen many children and adolescents of overweight adults suffer from their parents' obesity. As difficult as it can be to get children and adolescents to acknowledge the embarrassment they experience, they usually show tremendous relief once they are able to talk about their feelings. The offspring of obese adults are about 60 to 70 percent more likely to be overweight themselves. The suicide rate is much higher among overweight adolescents.

Think of the damage done to the self-esteem of someone who has repeatedly failed to lose weight on diet after diet. Consider the long-term effects that the many prejudices against obese individuals have on their self-esteem. There is no question that obesity has a detrimental psychological effect on people.

What kind of things do you say to yourself as you gorge on a bag of potato chips? What kind of messages creep into your psyche when you get a second helping even though your stomach is already full? Do you have kind words for yourself, or are you even aware of your thoughts? Most likely, when you treat your body unhealthily, you have detached yourself from your thinking system and feelings and are denying any thoughts or feelings with reckless abandon. The strategy of this book is to put you back in touch with those thoughts and feelings.

Next time you overeat, pause for a moment and listen to yourself. You will probably hear some very negative self-talk, statements such as, to quote a recent patient, "I'm a fat pig," or possibly, "I'm a weak idiot," or even, "What a slob I am."

In chapters 1 and 2, we talked at length about how your thoughts create your feelings and affect your brain. What kind of feelings do you suppose the above thoughts create for you? Even if you are not consciously aware of your self-talk, at some level you will experience the negative consequences of that kind of self-criticism.

Along the same line, what kind of message do you give to your body? When you look in the mirror, do you criticize what you see? Do you find yourself apologizing to others for the way you look? When people compliment you, do you try to contradict them? It is imperative that you begin to value your body right now. You must start where you are. Accept your body as it is. Only then can you start to change the way you treat it.

In your environment, there are plenty of opportunities to be criticized and ridiculed. Is there any reason to compound that with self-criticism? I think not.

Self-esteem is basically a concept that indicates how you feel about yourself and how you believe others see you. It is considered to be one of the best measures of well-being and overall mental health. Self-acceptance is a major part of this. It means acceptance of your thoughts, your feelings, your behavior, *and* your body.

The more you overeat, the more critical you are of yourself. The more you overeat, the more negative you feel as a result of that criticism. The more depressed you become, the more likely you are to numb yourself to your bad feelings by overeating. This negative feedback loop results in creating considerable shame and disgust with yourself. It's the proverbial vicious cycle.

Anger directed toward yourself is extremely damaging to your self-esteem. However, anger and extreme self-hatred are often experienced while watching yourself become obese. Is it possible that, in addition to experiencing anger toward yourself, you might feel anger toward those around you as they witness your weight gain?

You must begin to break this cycle by being kinder to yourself. Not only must you begin to treat yourself in a healthy manner, but you must also begin to suspend judgment of yourself if you have weak moments. Start reversing the cycle. This will not happen overnight. This program was never meant to be a quick fix. Each time you are able to avoid a food that does not fit into your new lifestyle, give yourself a pat on the back. Create a few positive self-talk statements so that you are tipping the scales gradually in a more positive direction. Examples of these statements would be, "I'm proud of myself for making the right choice," and "I am strong enough to avoid overeating." As you know, these thought patterns change not only your feelings, but your brain circuitry as well.

It's extremely important for you to begin to heighten your awareness of the link between your negative thoughts and your tendency to overeat. While we've looked at how your poor eating habits lead to low self-esteem, it is also likely that troubling thoughts unrelated to eating cause low self-esteem and result in eating to numb the negative feelings.

I recently had a patient, Richard, who retired from the military and is now a private consultant. I had him keep a diary of the negative, intrusive thoughts he was having about himself, noting the time of day and the circumstances under which they occurred. He found that many of his negative thoughts were accompanied by food urges.

The value of this assignment was threefold. First, he became more aware of how his negative thoughts about himself led to food cravings, and this awareness helped him to avoid indulging. Second, the repeated use of cognitive restructuring when these negative thoughts occurred, supported by using the self-hypnosis scripts, began to diminish his urges. Third, he began to explore what else accompanied the negative thoughts. Was his energy low? Was he tired? Could more exercise for the purpose of increasing energy level minimize the urges? Would more sleep lower the craving? Was he experiencing negative emotions toward others in his life that needed to be explored?

Obesity also causes difficulty in marriage. The frequency of sexual intimacy tends to be much lower when one of the partners is obese. Spouses of obese individuals often see them as less sexually attractive.

Without question, there are both physical and psychological consequences of being overweight. You hurt not only yourself, but potentially those around you. The costs of obesity on a national level are staggering. The sharp rise in health care costs is, in part, a consequence of obesity.

Self-hypnosis Script Five:
Sugar Avoidance

The majority of my patients have a difficult time avoiding sugar. Not only is the consumption of sugar very dangerous to your body, but it is probably the number one culprit in weight gain for most people. This segment is designed to develop your confidence in limiting your intake of refined sugar. There is also a sequence to develop an aversion to sugar.

In a nice, relaxed position, begin to breathe slowly and rhythmically, inhaling and exhaling, as you relax your shoulders and soften your belly.

Allow your body to breathe naturally and rhythmically.

Notice the support of the cushions beneath you as you begin to relax. Notice heaviness throughout your body as you become more and more relaxed.

Over the next several days, you will find yourself in many situations in which various forms of refined sugar will be available to you.

You know the situations, so begin to see yourself.

See yourself at home, out at your favorite restaurant, at work, at the grocery store, at the convenience store when you go in to pay for your gas—many situations—and the growing image you have of yourself is one of strength and confidence, feeling almost no desire for sugar.

Your head is held high, your shoulders are thrown back, and in your eye is a glimmer of hope.

You are feeling so good about yourself and your decision to limit refined sugar from your lifestyle.

That's right, you are going to limit refined sugar in your lifestyle because you know that sugar may be the number one culprit in lowering the quality of your life.

You will go as far as beginning to see sugar as almost lethal when ingested by your body.

You are becoming convinced that regardless of the situation, you will not allow yourself to overindulge in sweets.

Continue to develop this image of yourself feeling strong and having no desire for sugar.

With this image of yourself in your mind, take two or three nice, deep breaths.

With the first breath, just feel the confidence welling up in your chest.

With the next deep breath, feel the psychological strength centering in your body.

Take one more deep breath as the excitement courses through your veins—the excitement of knowing you will decrease your intake of sugar dramatically.

You are feeling so good about your decision to limit that old-fashioned and embarrassing habit of eating sugar.

You feel certain that you will be able to avoid refined sugar very often.

You are becoming more and more confident that you have the strength to avoid refined sugar on a regular basis.

To assist you in developing an aversion to sugar, you will be doing a rather difficult visualization. This visualization will help you to gain the strength to almost completely eliminate refined sugar.

You are going to see yourself seated at a large table covered with cakes, cookies, gallons of ice cream, candy, and even bowls of pure, granulated sugar. The table is piled high with sweets, and people are watching as you become increasingly embarrassed by your indulgence in sugar.

You are seeing people who are important to you watching you stuff your mouth with all the poisonous sugar food.

Your family, your friends, and your colleagues watch you as you poison your body with sugar, and you are feeling embarrassed.

That's right, you are literally becoming embarrassed as you stuff yourself with sugar.

You see yourself becoming—literally—fatter and fatter.

You see your clothing becoming tighter and tighter as you get fatter and fatter. The buttons on your shirt are popping off. The seams of your slacks are splitting.

You are imagining pure granulated sugar in your mouth.

It is almost repulsive and nauseating because you can hardly swallow.

As you hold this picture in your mind think:

For my body, sugar is poisonous.

I need my body to live.

I owe my body this respect and protection.

Anytime you are confronted with a decision to eat refined sugar, you will conjure up that image of yourself stuffing your body with sugar, and you will repeat:

For my body, sugar is poisonous.

I need my body to live.

I owe my body this respect and protection.

This will block almost any desire for sugar.

Imagine holding the remote control for your television. Press the "off" button and that negative image of you is gone.

Return now to the confident, strong, excited image, having no desire for sugar and feeling so good about yourself.

Just notice how much better that image of you feels.

That's right, you are feeling confident that you can control your craving for sugar.

It will become easier and easier to limit refined sugar because you want to live to see your children and grandchildren grow into healthy adults. You want to experience your life to the fullest.

You know there will be no situations in which you would allow yourself to overindulge in sugar.

You know that this desire for sugar reflects a malfunction in your brain, and not a real need to put sugar into your stomach. That's right, you are gradually changing the nature of your brain. Any urges for sugar are going to decrease steadily and become markedly less.

You are feeling very good about yourself, and you feel certain that you have the strength to avoid refined sugar when you choose.

You remember that sugar may be the number one culprit in lowering your quality of life and causing premature death.

With that thought in your mind, it will become easier and easier for you to avoid sugar. Your mind is changing your brain gradually so that you will no longer crave sugar.

Not because I am telling you, but because of the power of your subconscious mind you are going to be able to block almost all desire for sugar.

As you block the discomfort of craving sugar the urges become weaker and weaker and finally disappear.

Just allow yourself for a moment to imagine what sugar, that poisonous lethal habit, does to your body.

That image is going to help you to cope totally with any desire to eat sweets.

There will be no situation in which you will allow yourself to overindulge in sweets.

Visualize your head held high, your shoulders are thrown back, and you are feeling so good about your growing strength to avoid sugar.

You are becoming stronger and stronger and have almost no desire for sugar.

You really enjoy that image of strength and confidence. You will take that image of strength and confidence wherever you go.

Chapter Seven

Thinking about Your Behavior

"The demarcation between a positive and negative desire or action is not whether it gives you an immediate feeling of satisfaction but whether it ultimately results in positive or negative consequences."
—The Dalai Lama

Y ou probably remember behavioral psychologists Ivan Pavlov and B.F. Skinner from Psychology 101. These two took psychology from the intangible to the tangible, from brain to behavior, from the unobservable to the observable. They disagreed with Freud's premise that, if you dig deep into the minds of individuals and figure out what deep-seated issues from their past cause their difficulties, you will have sufficient knowledge to find the "cure." I agree with the behaviorists on this point: all the knowledge about childhood trauma isn't going to help you stop overeating.

However, even the psychoanalysts agree that when we catch ourselves in the moment—responding to urges to overeat—we can change our lives by changing our minds. This, in Freudian psychology, is about changing the subconscious mind to change your life. We have gone a big step further. We're also talking about changing your brain physically. And that is the real power—it's a physical brain change that supports and reinforces the mind changes that Freud and others wrote about. The changes take place because of your will to make them happen. This differentiates this program from anything Freudian or behaviorist, two schools of thought that don't recognize the will as a physical force. However, it has been proven that will is a physical force, and that using it to change your mind through cognitive restructuring causes your brain to change. In earlier chapters, we looked at the mind's influence regarding overeating and changing that behavior, and also how the mind changes the brain.

This chapter is about behavior. The behavior changes we're suggesting in this chapter will reinforce—and will be reinforced by—the changes you have made in your mind and your brain. It is a two-way street. We will be looking carefully at your actual behaviors—the ones that can cause or prevent weight gain—and how you think about these behaviors. This chapter presents mindful eating behavior. Acts of mindful eating behavior will reinforce your new thoughts and the changes in your brain—and, likewise, the thoughts and words from the self-hypnosis scripts will reinforce your mindful behavior. As Dr. Jeffrey M. Schwartz so succinctly states in his book *Dear*

Patrick: Letters to a Young Man, "Very recent research indicates that repeated thoughts and words may form nervous system interconnections that actually 'lay down tracks' for likely action." By repeating the thoughts about your behavior from this chapter, you will "lay down tracks" for the desired action. The more you are able to perform the desired action, the more your behavior or action will reinforce the good thoughts you have about eating. I believe there is room in your lifestyle changes for focusing on all aspects of your life, including your behavior, in order to lose weight.

I am going to review various strategies related to eating that you can incorporate into your lifestyle changes. These suggestions will involve actual observable behavior that you will begin to engage in to help you lose weight. Again, making these behavior changes in your life will reinforce and strengthen the changes you've made in your mind and brain.

"Eating behavior" is something that can be quantified, observed, and measured. When I use the word quantify, I am not referring to counting calories or fat grams, but to the actual observable behaviors that contribute to or deter weight loss, such as how fast you eat.

It is commonly agreed that the faster you eat, the more food you will consume before you experience the physical sensation of being full. In reality, one ought to stop eating just before feeling full—because food continues to expand when it enters your system and begins to digest. This is especially true with grains such as rice. By now, you have incorporated the thin attitude that food is fuel, and you are learning to stop eating once you feel full. You have also begun to acknowledge all feelings, and fullness is one of them.

There are several strategies that can aid in slowing the pace of food consumption. By employing these strategies, you will be able to experience fullness before you consume more food than is consistent with your new lifestyle. The nicest thing about eating more slowly is that you will enjoy your food more. Because you enjoy the food you eat, you will notice a sense of satisfaction, and it will be easier for you to stop at that point of satisfaction, rather than eat to the point of or beyond fullness.

Before you ever begin eating, take some time to notice the appearance of your food. Some meals are very attractive in appearance, especially if you are lucky enough to be a gourmet cook or to frequent gourmet restaurants. If you enjoy looking at cookbooks, you can understand the value of this suggestion. As you peruse your food visually, also acknowledge its aroma. This will begin to whet your appetite and get your digestive juices flowing. Once you pick up your fork, you are prepared to ingest your food; you have built up a healthy anticipation that sets you up for greater enjoyment of your meal. It is similar to going on a vacation. Anticipation is part of the enjoyment of traveling. The same can apply to the food you consume.

Once you do pick up your fork and begin eating, you will want to place your fork back on the table after each bite of food is placed in your mouth while you chew your food. This prevents you from refilling your fork and putting more food into your mouth before you chew and savor the current bite adequately. Putting your fork down and putting your hands in your lap results in slowing your pace of eating. This allows you to pay attention to the texture, the temperature, and the taste while the food is in your mouth, so that you savor every bite. By eating this way, you will be able to enjoy completely every bite of food that goes into your mouth. You want to make sure that you do not put another bite into your mouth until you have allowed the flavor of the current bite to fade away, allowing your taste buds to relax slightly so that you can experience the spectacular burst of flavor in your taste buds with your next bite of food. If you can allow yourself to taste the faded remnants of a bite of food, you are giving yourself the message that you do not need the continual pleasure and constant gratification of fast eating. If you eat so fast that you do not acknowledge these properties of your food, you probably will not enjoy your meal nearly as much. Without savoring your food you will not feel as satisfied. The more gastronomically satisfied you are, the less you will crave additional food after you have completed your meal or reached fullness. One of the reasons people who eat fast overeat is because they don't acknowledge, enjoy, or remember the taste of their food. Because the food is halfway down their throat before they actually acknowledge the taste, they have to put another bite in their mouth immediately. Thus, a vicious cycle begins, and I wonder if they ever really taste their food.

In his book, *Anger,* Thich Nhat Hanh recommends that we actually practice mindful eating, chewing food very carefully with full awareness and a lot of joy. He says we ought to "appreciate that it is wonderful to be sitting here chewing like this, not worrying about anything. When we eat mindfully, we are not chewing or eating our anger, our anxiety or our projects." Hanh also recommends chewing until the food is almost liquefied because you experience the flavors more intensely. Another benefit of chewing your food extensively is that it is already partially digested when it arrives in your stomach, making digestion much easier and more effective.

Since I mentioned gourmet cooking, I would like to add that, contrary to popular belief, most gourmet cooks are not overweight. One of the main reasons is that they eat as Thich Nhat Hanh suggests. Also, gourmet cooks do not cook gourmet meals every night. However, when they do cook a gourmet meal, they plan ahead and, beginning the day before or the day of the big meal, they limit their intake in anticipation. As you know and we have discussed, food tastes better when you are hungry. This idea of planning ahead might also be used for special occasions like holidays.

Do you derive pleasure from preparing your food? If you take your time and enjoy the preparation, you are more likely to eat slowly as you enjoy the fruits of your labor.

Another way of slowing down the pace of eating is to drink water with your meal. It is not necessary to drink after every bite, but it is advisable to drink at least an eight-ounce glass of water with each meal. This is also advisable because it aids in digestion and contributes to a full feeling sooner.

How much food have you consumed while standing at the refrigerator door, the pantry door, standing over the stove cooking, or during clean up? How many meals have you consumed behind the wheel of your motor vehicle? So many of the mothers of small children I work with talk about eating the leftovers from their children's plates. You can begin to believe you will stop that behavior and never again eat your children's leftovers. It is an unhealthy habit and your decision right here, right now, will allow you never to do this again.

It is probably obvious that, except in very rare situations, I am very much opposed to fast food, especially French fries and other fried foods loaded with trans fat. Many fast food restaurants are serving healthy alternatives now so that, if you must eat on the run, you can make a healthy decision. However, eating while driving or riding in a car is inappropriate behavior. Bottom line: food is to be consumed while sitting at a table. Eating should be given your undivided attention.

We live in very fast-paced society, and because of this we often multitask. Examples of multitasking are eating while driving, reading, watching TV, or talking on the telephone. Multitasking leads to mindless, or semiconscious, eating— eating without savoring the food. Often we don't realize how much is consumed and, ultimately, we overeat.

Of course, we all know that if no one sees you eating, it doesn't count. Yeah, right! It is probably a good idea to try to consume most of your food around like-minded people. They help make us more accountable.

If, however, you often consume food alone, there is one danger to consider. Because you are eating alone, you may not feel the need to set the table and sit down to eat. It is important not to stand at the refrigerator and eat, because you may just dive into one thing after another with little awareness of how much you have consumed. Instead, fill a plate appropriately and sit down to eat. Don't fall into the trap of grazing or foraging.

Occasionally, as a side dish or light lunch, I will eat whole-grain crackers and mozzarella cheese. It is a good idea to get out only the number of crackers you want to eat, slice off the serving of cheese, and put the rest away. Before I changed my lifestyle, I would leave out the box of crackers and the package of cheese, and, before I knew it I had consumed three or four servings of each—at least twice as much as I had originally intended. A similar pattern often occurs with a can of peanuts: in a few minutes, you may consume as many as three or four 170-calorie servings. Set yourself up for success by measuring your portions.

Another way of controlling your weight is to consider the time of day when you consume food. David Kirsch, author of *Sound Mind Sound Body*, considers the time between 9:00 p.m. and 6:00 a.m. to be the "red zone." He suggests that eating during this time tends to be mood related rather than hunger related. By this time, your activity level has slowed down, so the digestive process will slow as well, and you are more likely to gain weight. Eating during these hours also impedes good sleep.

A deterrent to weight gain that seems to have an ever-so-subtle effect on overweight individuals is to have them lie down on the floor to feel the fat. It's possible to look in a mirror without seeing the fat, and whether it is the clothing you wear that camouflages the extra weight or simply denial that causes a distorted body image, some people don't see it. However, lying on the floor, on your stomach, your side, and your back, you cannot very easily deny what excess fat feels like on your body. This is another sensory input to connect you to reality.

Whether slowing the pace of eating, eating mindfully, eating in a timely manner, or simply paying attention to the appearance of your food, you will find that these strategies will not only enhance the enjoyment of eating but will also lead to weight loss. There is so much at your disposal to help you to lose weight. I hope that this chapter will help you to employ more of these resources.

Self-hypnosis Script Six:
Slowing the Pace of Eating

This segment is designed to help you not only slow down the pace of your eating but enjoy your food more. You can employ the strategy of a gourmet by eating slowly and savoring each bite that goes into your mouth. As you know, food tastes much better when you are pleasantly hungry. Begin this session by getting yourself into a relaxed, meditative frame of mind.

Focus your attention on your breathing.

Do not alter the natural rhythm of your breathing, and begin to notice the rising and falling of your chest.

Notice the sensations of the inhalation and exhalation on the supple tissue of your nostrils.

Continue the relaxed rhythmic breathing for two to three minutes as you prepare for the self-hypnosis script.

When you do begin to visualize—and even if you read—you will initially visualize what you have read with your eyes closed; do not think of visualizing with your eyes, but, rather, imagine the visualizations appearing within your mind, in its open space.

Try focusing on a point between and just above the eyes.

Imagine that you are looking at this point from a short distance, further back.

Picture yourself preparing to eat and feeling comfortably hungry.

If you are filling your own plate, you probably have a plate that is about twelve inches in diameter.

Before you begin to fill your plate, you are going to imagine the plate shrinking down to only about ten inches in diameter, the size of a large salad plate.

If it was twelve inches at first and now it is ten inches, it is now roughly one-third smaller in size.

That's right, one-third smaller—that's how it calculates.

Quite spontaneously, and with the force of your will, you are going to begin taking smaller portions whenever you fill your own plate.

If your food is being served to you, or if you have filled your own plate, you have a dinner plate in front of you that has a healthy meal on it.

Before you begin to eat, fold your hands in your lap, and notice the food on your plate.

As you look at it, carefully notice the appearance and aroma of your food.

When you pick up your fork, you will take a bite of food that fits comfortably in your mouth, probably a little smaller than the bites you used to take.

As you begin to chew your food, notice the taste, the texture, and the temperature of that bite of food.

As you are chewing the bite—and you will chew it at least a dozen times—you have placed your fork back on your plate and put your hands back in your lap.

After two or three more bites of food, eaten in just the same way, you will take a drink of water.

While you eat, notice the sensations in your stomach as it begins to fill.

As you are eating, you are noticing how good your food tastes.

If you are eating with others, make sure that, when you speak, you do not speak with food in your mouth.

You are staying ever mindful of the fact that you are eating, and you are eating to live, not living to eat.

As you learn to eat more slowly and enjoy the food you are eating, you will find that you have a full feeling in your stomach much sooner than usual.

You are learning to be mindful and to pay attention to every bite that goes into your mouth.

You savor and enjoy each bite.

You savor and enjoy each bite until the flavor of that bite fades.

You will pause, ever so briefly, after each bite so you get to enjoy that spectacular burst of flavor with each new bite of food.

Because you enjoy each bite of food, you feel very satisfied and find that you need much less food to satisfy your taste buds.

You also begin to notice a full feeling in your stomach much sooner than usual. As you begin to feel the full feeling in your stomach much sooner than usual, you will simply stop eating.

In a very interesting way, because of the strength of your visualization, you will stop eating before you are completely full.

Once the food is in your stomach, it will begin to expand slightly as it is digested and mixes with your digestive juices. Because of your awareness of the full feeling in your stomach much sooner than usual, you will begin to leave food behind on your plate.

That's right. Quite spontaneously, without willpower, you will begin to leave food behind on your plate.

It will be interesting to you to see yourself learning to listen to your body, learning to leave food behind on your plate when you feel full.

You will begin to see the food that is left behind on your plate when you are pleasantly full as belonging in the refrigerator as leftovers, or in the garbage can.

If you consume any food once you are full, you are treating yourself like a garbage can.

That is not part of your lifestyle.

Once you are pleasantly full, you will put your fork down for the last time and stop eating.

You are pleasantly satisfied with no desire to overeat, no desire to overeat.

You are learning to listen to your body, and you notice how you feel satisfied with less food.

You simply notice how soon you feel comfortably full and content with no desire to overeat.

You will be thrilled and delighted at how completely satisfied you are with considerably less food. That's right— much less food, much more satisfied.

Each time you eat in this manner, you are strengthening the neural pathways in your brain that lead to a healthy lifestyle, and you are shrinking those pathways that allowed you to eat too hurriedly and too much.

That's right—you are completely satisfied and happy to stop eating.

You see yourself feeling very confident that you can and will stop eating very happily when you feel full.

You are so excited that you can now stop eating when your stomach is full and feel no desire to overeat.

Chapter Eight

The Importance of Exercise

"Any diet book that claims permanent weight loss
without exercise is counterfeit."
—Covert Baily

A recent issue of the *American Psychological Association
Monitor* on self-care for psychologists began with an
article on health suggesting that "if you do just one
thing make it exercise." Throughout this book, I have attempt-
ed repeatedly to broaden the focus from simple weight loss to
general self-care. It is my belief that if you avoid the narrow
focus of weight loss as your primary goal you will lessen the
stress and obsession with weight and potentially lose more
weight.

In this chapter, I have chosen not to emphasize exercise for
the purpose of losing weight because so much is already written
about it—and it is so obvious. In order to lose weight, you have

to exercise. I believe that if you look at the many other benefits of exercise and take the pressure off exercising just to lose weight, you might be more inclined to begin exercising. You have associated previous failed attempts to exercise with failure to lose weight. This time, you will exercise for new—and better—reasons. With this new attitude and approach to exercise, you may find a motivation that you lacked in the past. That is what we'll work to accomplish in this chapter.

Most diet books and programs encourage exercise to lose weight. Most of my patients have owned several of these books. Still, upon coming to my office, most of them had never adhered to a regular exercise program for an extended period of time. Some diet books have page after page explaining the physiology of exercise to aid in weight loss. They include equations of fat-burning physiology, calorie counting/burning models, lean body charts, body fat ideals, and so on. Still, most people don't exercise regularly. Obviously, the benefit of weight loss is not enough to motivate people to adhere to a regular exercise program.

According to the U.S. Department of Health and Human Services, most Americans do not participate regularly in physical activity. In a fairly recent report, DHHS reports that only 15 percent of adults participate in vigorous physical exercise "three times a week for at least twenty minutes." Of those individuals who do start an exercise program, 50 percent will drop out within six months.

So what can possibly be the formula for convincing overweight people to exercise? In my program, I have included various strategies. It is important to find a match with your personality. Aerobic exercise alone is probably not sufficient to speed up your metabolism. Some sort of resistance training is also necessary in order to maintain sufficient muscle mass. In addition to building muscle, you also strengthen your bones.

Many of my patients lament the inevitability of weight gain because of slowed metabolic rate with aging. A study by Tzankhoff and Norris shows that the slowing of metabolism is due not to aging but to the body losing muscle mass. Larger, heavier muscles continue to burn calories, even when your body is otherwise at rest. If you are not doing some type of resistance training or muscle-building exercises, your muscle mass will decrease, resulting in a slower metabolic rate. Therefore, the excuse that weight gain is unavoidable because of aging is simply untrue.

Weight lifting can also benefit the cardiovascular system. If you lift at a slow and consistent rate, you will begin to notice an increase in your heart rate. Weight lifting also improves your body's ability to process insulin and distribute glucose through-out your system. Strong muscles also provide better support to your skeletal system, another vital benefit, especially for the aging body.

One of the suggestions I make is for my clients to incorpo-rate exercise into their daily routine. Some of the obvious things you can do are taking the stairs instead of the elevator, parking farther from your destination, and cleaning your house and car rather than hiring someone else to do it. Do your own gardening and yard work. If you have a dog, a regular walk would benefit both of you. Regarding sex: make your sexual intimacy more active and playful.

Another benefit of exercise is that it enhances other endeavors by increasing both your physical and mental acuity. When I was working on my PhD, I always tried to run before an important exam. I saw the benefit as twofold: first, it eased my tension and anxiety and thus put me in a better frame of mind to take the test. Second, a good run sharpens the mind because it enhances delivery of oxygen to cerebral tissue.

I have also had patients who want to quit smoking begin exercising. Again, exercise provides an excellent way to release the tension related to cigarette cravings. They claim that it calms them and diminishes the craving.

Exercise can also be a way of spending time with your spouse or other significant person. If you make a commitment to each other, it might increase the likelihood of exercising. There may be days when one of you is less motivated, and encouragement from the other will really help to keep you on track.

I have had several patients who began exercising as part of a goal to raise money for a charity. One of my patients recently lost her mother after a lengthy battle with breast cancer. Her mother's death motivated her to do a walk to raise money for breast cancer. A good friend recently entered a training program for a triathlon to raise money for the Leukemia Society. The event consists of just under a one-mile swim, a twenty-six-mile bike ride, and just over a six-mile run. A worthy cause for exercising can be motivating. Training for something like this may take a long time, which may result in exercise becoming a habit. Once a habit is ingrained and the benefits become apparent, the odds are that it will become a permanent lifestyle change.

I have walked with many of my patients during therapy sessions. You may be able to carry out one of your meetings while walking. Find a friend with whom you regularly meet to talk and try to have your conversation while walking. Walking around the zoo, a museum, or botanical garden might enhance the enjoyment of your exercise. If possible, walk or ride your bike rather than driving to work or to run errands. All of these choices are part of the continuous decision making that losing weight requires.

When discussing lifestyle changes as opposed to dieting in chapter 3, I suggested the concept of a long-term life endeavor. Just like changing your lifestyle regarding eating, exercise must also be considered a permanent lifestyle change. You cannot exercise only until the weight is lost and then stop and expect the weight to stay off.

A *Wichita Eagle* newspaper article by Karen Shideler explores what keeps the fitness experts going on bad-attitude days. Working out first thing in the morning is one of the experts' suggestions. I personally used to try to fit my workout in either at noon or after work. However, on too many days something would come up and I would miss my workout. If I set my alarm an hour ahead of time in the morning, I felt I had more control over making sure I had enough time for my workout.

Another reason I work out in the morning is that it sets a good tone for the remainder of the day. The stillness and solitude of early morning is appealing to me. When I first began exercising early, I could count on a predictable opposition from some place in my mind. I had to tell myself as I was setting my alarm the night before that I was going to get out of bed no matter what thoughts found their way to the forefront. I made a commitment to get up early, whether some part of my mind felt like it or not. Regardless of the time of day when you choose to exercise, you may have to use this reasoning.

As you learned in chapters 1 and 2, my decision to get up deepened the grooves in my neural pathways that said "get up" and not the ones that said "stay in bed." This discipline became a part of me. It became a habit. Now, I cannot imagine sleeping in when I have made a decision to get up early.

For people who have trouble getting up early, it's important to remember that the anguish of getting out of bed lasts only a few seconds. Once you are out of bed and your feet are on the floor, the battle is usually won. Don't touch that snooze button! Or if you do, you can use this time—while fudging on your duty to get up—to think about the ideas presented in the self-hypnosis scripts in this book and help set your day in the right direction from the very beginning. You are in a special state of consciousness at those moments, not unlike a meditative state of mind.

Another expert suggests varying your workout. This has always worked well for me. On weekends, I try to walk eighteen holes on the golf course. I lift weights two to three times per week. I practice yoga two to three times per week. I walk my dog two to three times per week. I try to play tennis occasionally. This may sound like a lot of exercise, but, some days, I may lift weights for only forty-five minutes and, later in the day, walk my dog for thirty minutes. I manage to do this while working full time, too. Not everyone can expect to do this much, but I have worked into this weekly pattern over several years of commitment. You can simply discover what you can do over several years, and you may surprise yourself. The more exercise you do, the more you find yourself capable of doing. Don't let the appearance of my very busy exercise schedule deter you from doing this. I don't perceive it as a burden or as being "very busy"—it is just how I live. And your new lifestyle will become just how you live.

Other suggestions from the experts include goal setting and working out with a friend. Shideler also suggests you listen to your self-talk. Are you really just making excuses, but telling yourself they are good reasons not to exercise? Promise yourself that you will do something almost every day. It doesn't have to be a triathlon event, but something—anything—that fits where you can start now and later, something that fits what you can envision for the future. That vision will change for the better over time. Don't necessarily plan to take a day off, because you know that, inevitably, there will be days when you simply cannot fit in exercise. Once you are in the habit of exercising regularly, you may want to give yourself a day off occasionally and not feel guilty about it. But, on other days, even if you jump rope for ten minutes in the garage at midnight, it is better than nothing. Those short workouts do add up and help keep you from letting the time between workouts extend too long. The longer your break in exercise, the easier it is to blow it off the next day.

One of the reasons exercise adherence is so low is that the realized benefits do not kick in soon enough. Once the many benefits are felt, though, you are more likely to stick with your program. Regardless of your age, it is not too soon to consider the research indicating that older adults who have sustained exercise programs long-term report greater life satisfaction, due in large part to greater self-sufficiency.

The psychological benefits of weight loss occur not only because of weight reduction but for other reasons as well. Millions of Americans suffer from varying levels of anxiety and depression. Countless research studies show a strong correlation between exercise and a reduction in anxiety and depression. Although exercise ought to be performed regularly, results can be realized even after just one workout session.

The physiological changes, such as increased cerebral blood flow, reduced muscle tension, changes in brain neurotransmitters (endorphins and norepinephrine), increased maximal oxygen consumption, and delivery of oxygen to cerebral tissues are all potential reasons for lowering anxiety and depression and, ultimately, enhancing psychological well-being.

In chapter 6, we talked about how being overweight negatively impacts your self-esteem. The weight itself and the negative self-talk combine to take an extreme toll on how you feel about yourself. Research has shown that exercise can increase self-esteem significantly, and that is especially true for individuals who have very low self-esteem. The increase in self-esteem is not just a result of weight loss or improved fitness. Other factors such as socialization, feelings of increased physical competence, enhanced feelings of control, and goal attainment all combine to increase self-esteem.

As you have seen in this book—and will continue to see—many of the self-hypnosis scripts involve development of very positive images about yourself. It has been proven that seeing positive images of yourself produces the brain chemical endorphin. Endorphins are considered our natural pain-killers and often bring feelings of euphoria or pleasure when active in the brain. For those of you who eat to comfort yourself, the endorphins produced by positive self-imagery and exercise will begin to replace the role of food as your buffer against the inevitable pain of being human. As mentioned earlier, exercise also produces endorphins—runners sometimes refer to the high they get while running, and after the run, from the endorphins. Other forms of exercising can produce it, too.

Crystal, who has maintained a healthy lifestyle for quite some time, called recently to update me on her progress. She was especially excited about how her exercise program is giving her more self-esteem and helping her with her food choices. She told me about going for a three-mile walk the previous morning, then going in to work to find someone had brought homemade brownies and left them in the break room. For a split second, she considered taking one. Then, she immediately told herself that after all her effort to walk there was no way she was going to blow it for a brownie. She could see how her exercise was helping her stick to her lifestyle changes.

There is also an accumulating body of research indicating that exercise may help reduce insomnia. Insomnia affects approximately one-third of the adult population with negative side effects, such as decreased productivity, increased mortality, irritability, and psychiatric disturbances. If you exercise regularly, the aforementioned physiological responses, the calming effects exercise has on mood, as well as the physical fatigue it produces, all enhance the body's ability to sleep.

Our lives are very fast-paced and, as J. Kornfield suggests in *A Path with Heart*, we are addicted to speed. "Technological society pushes us to increase the pace of our productivity and the pace of our lives...In a society that almost demands life at double time, speed addictions numb us to our own experience. In such a society it is almost impossible to settle into our bodies or stay connected with our hearts." Exercise may provide a respite from that fast pace, as well as an opportunity to settle into our bodies.

The idea that exercise provides a break from the fast pace of life may seem contradictory. If you can rethink your exercise and see it as an opportunity to get away from it all, you can learn to put yourself into a meditative state. Turn your awareness inward and begin learning to connect with your body. Work toward clearing your mind of the chatter of your day. Look at exercise as a reward or time-out from the hustle and bustle of your day.

Exercise has also been associated with increases in cognitive functioning. This may be due in part to the physiological benefits of cerebral blood flow, maximal oxygen consumption, and delivery to cerebral tissue caused by exercise.

Additional psychological benefits of exercise may include an increase in academic performance, assertiveness, emotional stability, internal locus of control, positive body image, self-control, sexual satisfaction, and work efficiency. Absenteeism at work, alcohol abuse, anger, confusion, headaches, phobias, psychotic behavior, and tension all potentially decrease as a result of exercise.

These are by no means the only benefits of exercise. Many individuals report their own esoteric benefits. Once you begin to exercise, you may discover additional benefits. Remember, the reason many people stop exercising is that they have not persevered long enough to realize the benefits.

There are very few, if any, good reasons for not exercising, and numerous poor excuses. The three most commonly cited "reasons" are lack of time, lack of energy, and lack of motivation.

Lack of time is undoubtedly more perception than reality and comes down to one's priorities. If you have time to watch TV, read the newspaper, talk on the phone, read a book, or shop, you have time to exercise.

The idea that you are too tired to exercise is contradicted by research that shows that regular exercise actually increases energy levels. Fatigue may be stress related, and research also indicates that regular exercise may be the most efficient and reliable method of relieving stress.

Your lack of motivation is probably related to your attitude toward exercise. As Ian K. Smith suggests in *The Take Control*

Diet, it is not a competitive attitude, but a "determination to submit your body to a physical stress that in the long run will improve your physical stature, overall health, and mental energy."

Exercise is one of the best ways to enhance your awareness of your body and to develop a more intimate relationship with your body. Without exercising, you run the risk of ignoring the subtle signals that are constantly emerging from your body. This may blunt your awareness of who you are physically, making it especially difficult to experience your body as a source of pleasure.

You are now aware of the countless benefits of exercise other than weight loss, and have at your disposal an arsenal of reasons to exercise that should greatly enhance your motivation. You will begin to exercise for the experience itself. In the next chapter, we will look at the body as a source of pleasure— which should boost your motivation to exercise even more.

Self-hypnosis Script Seven:
Exercise

It is a well-documented fact that moderate amounts of exercise usually energize you. I know most people believe that exercise uses up energy. This segment is designed to help you begin to internalize the sense of exhilaration you can get from the energy gained through exercise.

Sit quietly and comfortably.

Inhale softly, exhale gently.

Inhale softly, exhale gently.

Let your body drift and rest easily.

Let go of all the thoughts of your day, thoughts of past and future, memories, and plans.

Just be right here, right now.

You are pleasantly relaxed, ready to begin creating a positive mindset toward exercise.

You are beginning to believe that you can exercise regularly and feel good about yourself for doing it.

Begin by bringing up a memory from your past in which you felt exhilarated.

Picture a time in your life when you were very excited about something.

You are jumping up and down, clapping and hugging someone.

You may have just received some great news.

Now that you have the memory and feeling of exhilaration fixed in your mind, picture yourself putting on your exercise clothing.

You find yourself looking forward to your exercise and the accompanying feeling of exhilaration.

It will become important to you to exercise almost every day, and the decision to do so will become easier and easier.

If brief moments of indecision enter your mind, you simply let go of them and go back to looking forward to the good feelings you will have as a result of exercising.

You know that you will feel a sense of accomplishment along with an increase in your self-esteem.

You will feel energized, and your mood will be elevated.

Regardless of the circumstances, you will be motivated to exercise on those days you are scheduled to exercise.

And, of course, you know that almost every day is an exercise day.

You will find time for exercise on a consistent, regular basis and feel so good about yourself.

You will begin to notice that your exercise lowers your anxiety and tension and creates a lovely, pleasurable sensation within your body.

Just notice for a few seconds how good it feels to see yourself exercising and realizing all of the tremendous benefits of exercise.

Go back to that feeling of exhilaration, just enjoy the effects and relax.

You are strengthening the neural pathways in your brain that will motivate you to exercise.

You are going to be thrilled and delighted at how your subconscious mind simply blocks any discouraging thoughts or poor excuses not to exercise.

Each time you make a decision to exercise it is going to begin to feel very natural to you.

Picture yourself doing your favorite exercise, whether it is walking, running, yoga, swimming, or bicycling.

You are seeing yourself exercising and feeling very good about your decision to exercise.

You are feeling very confident that you will begin exercising regularly.

Your visualization of yourself in a more slender form as a result of exercising is very exciting to you.

That image alone is going to give you more motivation to exercise on a regular basis.

You are feeling very excited that regular exercise will become a permanent part of your lifestyle.

Chapter Nine

The Body as a Pleasure Source

"It is also helpful to realize that this very body that we have, that's sitting right here, right now...with its aches and its pleasures is exactly what we need to be fully human, fully awake, fully alive."
—Pema Chodren, Tibetan Buddhist Nun

On the way home from work, I drive by a house where a rather portly gentleman is often outside working on his car. It appears that he spends several hours a week washing, waxing, cleaning the engine, and detailing the inside of his car. Yet, it is so obvious that he is neglecting his body. He gets such pleasure out of manicuring his car and, I suspect, great pride from the results. Yet, he appears to lack pride in his body.

JoAnn, a patient of mine, came to me for help losing weight. She indicated that she was what she considered a neat freak. She spent well over an hour a day vacuuming, dusting, and scrubbing, but not one minute exercising. She was deriving pleasure from her clean house—but might she not find more pleasure in life through a healthy body? Granted, she did get some exercise cleaning, but not of the intensity necessary to lose weight. JoAnn pledged to herself that she would not do any house cleaning until she had exercised for at least thirty minutes. She found that this worked very well for her. Do you see your body as a source of pleasure? Do you treat it as something from which you seek pleasure? I do not think you can separate the way you treat your body from the way you treat yourself—or, for that matter, people in general. Seeing your body as a potential source of pleasure should help you to value and nurture it more carefully and attentively. It may just be a whole new lease on life for you.

I encourage my patients to see their bodies as the physical plants through which they experience their lives. "You cannot do a single thing," writes Deepak Chopra, "from falling in love to uttering a prayer to metabolizing a molecule of sucrose, without affecting everything that you are." Yoga author Rodney Yee refers to the body as the "tool for living, the instrument through which the music of life is played."

Both of these quotes reinforce the importance of your body in your life. Your body is like a temple; it is often referred to as the home of the spirit. It is the physical plant through which we experience our lives. The extent to which you want to enjoy and experience your life to its fullest will depend greatly on how physically fit you are. How physically fit you are will depend, among other things, upon the kind of relationship you have with your body. Have you ever considered a relationship with your body?

Like most overweight people, it is very possible that you made an unconscious decision to subordinate your body at some point in your life. Ram Dass in *Still Here* describes how he did just that until, because he ignored the warning signs, he suffered a stroke.

One reason people in our modern society have such a difficult time experiencing their bodies as a source of pleasure is that they rarely experience their bodies at all. Can one experience pleasure in one's body without settling into it? Probably not.

Many of my patients tell me their only source of pleasure is eating. My first response is to ask them to think about how it feels to wake up in the morning and have a good, spontaneous stretch. If they have a cat or a dog, I tell them to watch their pet the next time it stretches. Can you tell how much pleasure is derived from the stretch? Often, I have my patients reach for the ceiling right there in my office and stretch, stretch, stretch. I can tell that it feels good to them.

This is a good way to begin to see the simple, subtle pleasure you can derive from your body and begin to think of ways to experience your body as a source of pleasure.

The paradox, of course, is that you cannot overeat and experience pleasure in your body. There may be an extremely brief period of pleasure as the food is ingested; however, it is often accompanied by intense guilt, not to mention the pain of poisoning your body, and the extreme discomfort of being too full.

So many of my patients have related stories to me about seeing themselves in a mirror and thinking, "Who is that person?" They say they've been able to deny the poor shape into which they've allowed their bodies to grow. The attitude some people express borders on self-loathing. It will not be easy to treat your body well if you are repulsed by the sight of it or if it is a source of shame rather than pleasure.

If you were at your ideal weight, would it be easier to imagine your body as a source of pleasure? Do you remember your body being a source of pleasure for you in the past? Did you derive pleasure from your appearance? How about the photo of you in your wedding dress or your football uniform from many years ago?

The notion of one's body being a source of pleasure might be considered a taboo subject for many. The reason for this may be that, when we think of our bodies in this context, it is most often in a sexual sense. Sexual pleasure is undoubtedly one of the more common and important ways in which we seek pleasure through our bodies; however, it is only one of many. Sexual pleasure is a highly appropriate source of pleasure. We are sexual beings from birth until death. That pleasure ought to be encouraged and applauded within a healthy context.

However, there is no question that sexual pleasure is greatly diminished for the obese, as well as their partners. A frequently asked question is, "Will my sex drive improve if I lose weight?" The answer is almost unquestionably YES! This improvement occurs for several reasons.

First, by losing weight, you will become more physically fit. When you are more physically fit, your body's sensitivity to touch is heightened. The muscle response to sensitivity is much greater. An orgasm, in a physical sense, is not a purely genital, physical response. If you are truly physically fit, you will experience orgasm throughout much of your body, even though much of the stimulation that ultimately results in orgasm is in the genital area. Believe me, I've been fit and not-so-fit, and the sexual experience is dramatically different in a fit body.

Second, sexual pleasure often involves visual stimulation as well. I know many individuals who are embarrassed by their physical appearance and refuse to have sex unless it is dark. Your physical appearance may not be as much of an issue for your partner as it is for you. If you don't feel good about the appearance of your body, you may have a difficult time deriving sexual pleasure from it. A college professor once said that truly pleasurable, intimate sex occurs when you are "eyeball to eye-ball" with your partner.

Unfortunately, it is often assumed that your partner is responsible for your sexual pleasure. I strongly disagree with this. For a sexual experience to be most fulfilling, your own involvement, as well as your partner's, will be essential. If you are repulsed by the appearance and feel of your body, how motivated are you going to be to participate in your own pleasure? So, to reiterate, your feelings about your body and the fitness of your body are going to influence the degree of pleasure you derive from sex significantly.

Sex is only one of many ways your body can be a source of pleasure. Being physically fit can contribute to a myriad of pleasurable physical experiences as well.

If you have never been a runner, you cannot imagine the physical pleasure experienced from a good, long run. The feeling of fatigue creates an incredibly wonderful, paradoxical pleasure, not to mention the endorphin release that many refer to as runner's high.

Yesterday I was playing tennis and hit a series of good backhands. I was working on being more compact and smooth with my swing. After about six to eight backhands in a row, I began to feel an incredibly pleasing rhythm and muscle burn throughout my glutes, quads, and hamstrings. I also felt great pleasure from the rhythm of the movements. If I were struggling to catch my breath or experiencing lower back pain because of carrying around thirty to forty extra pounds, I don't believe I would ever have noticed the sweet, paradoxical experience of muscle burn, or the pleasant rhythm of my body at work.

Weight lifting provides opportunity for pleasure as well. This occurs sometimes as a result of the termination of muscle burn. If you are a golfer, you have probably had the rare experience of hitting a ball perfectly. That feeling resonates throughout your entire body.

Yoga probably provides, for me, the most dramatic sense of pleasure through exercising my body. In addition to providing intense pleasure, it is, in my opinion, the most youth-sustaining exercise available. It develops not only greater flexibility, but better balance, posture, and strength as well. If you have ever observed an older person walking, probably more obvious than their appearance is their shortened stride, stiff gait, and poor posture. Yoga will help to prevent all of these.

I have been practicing yoga for several years, and I cannot adequately describe how pleasurable the experience can be. It is a feeling of great accomplishment to hold a difficult balance pose longer than ever before, or to extend a stretch an eighth of an inch farther. It creates a tremendous sense of connectedness with every cell in my body. It is as if everything comes together—my breathing, heartbeat, the muscles required to sustain the pose, and quiet mind—allowing the experience to occur unhampered by competition or expectation. The balancing also creates a feeling of connectedness to the earth. The purpose of yoga is to create symmetry and balance in your body, your mind, and, ultimately, your life. In addition to suspending any competitive urge or expectation, yoga connects you to the present moment. We don't know about the future and the past is already gone, so we have only this precious moment. There is no preoccupation with painful memories of your past or anxieties about your future.

Although I speak of yoga as a pathway to experiencing your body as a source of pleasure, it also provides an excellent method of connecting your mind, body, and spirit. Deepak Chopra states that "at every stage of spiritual growth, the greatest ally you have is your body."

Thich Nhat Hanh suggests that we need to overcome the duality that views the mind and body as entirely separate. What happens to your mind happens to your body. Yoga provides an opportunity to bridge that separation. It may also heighten your awareness of how the food you consume affects not only your body but your mind as well. It may help you to become more attuned to the idea that you are what you eat.

Yoga is also one form of exercise that, after a rather short time of practicing, you get pulled into. It is not like an exercise you have to talk yourself into. After yoga, you feel relaxed and energized, and you cannot wait for that experience again. You look forward to your next yoga class.

If you think of your body as a source of pleasure and view it as a continuation from little to optimum pleasure, the low end of the continuum could actually be painful. Consider something as rudimentary as breathing. For me, a deep, full breath of fresh air is a source of pleasure. For someone who is obese and in poor physical health, trying to breathe after walking up a flight of stairs can be painful.

If you are at the lower end of the continuum, consider what you are missing. How can a person become obese at the expense of the privilege of experiencing pleasure through their body? It may be important to try to gain a greater understanding of how your body became a source of displeasure. Can you understand how missing out on a tremendous opportunity for pleasure through your body detracts from your overall sense of contentment in life?

Consider things like the pleasure of a tennis match with your granddaughter. How wonderful does a walk in the park with your friends sound? What about a wonderfully stimulating sexual encounter with your spouse? In *Open to Desire*, Mark

Epstein suggests that "our indefatigable pursuit of pleasure keeps us doing some awfully strange things." If eating is one of your few pleasures, you may be doing one of these so-called "strange" things. I sincerely hope you can begin to look forward to finding more pleasure through your body in healthy ways. A different mindset about the body you inhabit and what you might gain from it can open up vast new experiences for you.

The body is the means by which we enact our attitudes, values, and beliefs. I invite you to begin to see the maintenance of your body as a spiritual duty. Begin this duty as an act of love and compassion toward yourself and all of humankind.

Self-hypnosis Script Eight:
Changing Your Focus

You will begin to notice that this self-hypnosis strategy is capable of focusing your mind on what you are for, rather than what you are against.

In a very comfortable setting, begin to take some nice, deep, rhythmic breaths. With each inhalation, begin to clear your mind of all the thoughts of your day and simply begin to relax.

You are becoming more and more relaxed and calm with each exhalation.

You are finding yourself in a very pleasant meditative state. Begin to notice how calm, relaxed, and ready you are to receive your messages.

It is true that overeating or eating the wrong kinds of food is poisonous, and you are against this, but your emphasis is upon your commitment to protect your health.

That's right—your emphasis is upon your commitment to value and protect your body.

Because of your commitment to your health, it is going to begin to feel natural as you begin to protect your body against the poison and pollution of overeating.

When you make this commitment to respect your body, there is a power within you to make radical changes in your eating behavior.

You are not going to be excessively nervous, nor will you be tense.

Your emphasis on what you are for will begin to make your lifestyle changes feel very natural to you.

You are beginning to see your lifestyle changes as something you are doing for yourself.

You are not depriving yourself, but moving toward giving your body more respect and pleasure.

Only an overeater sees these lifestyle changes as deprivation.

You are truly giving up your old identity as an overeater and accepting the identity of a normal, healthy eater.

A normal, healthy eater does not feel deprived.

Even if you have been an overeater for many years, you are going to give up that old-fashioned and embarrassing identity.

Since your focus is upon your health rather than overeating, you begin to spend your time thinking more about your health.

In many situations, you will find that, when confronted with a lifestyle choice, your thoughts move toward healthy choices.

Your powerful thoughts and the force of your will are going to begin changing the circuitry of your brain and it will become easier and easier to make healthy choices.

That's right—it seems very natural for you to choose a healthy body over unhealthy food choices.

You find yourself protecting your body naturally, treating it with kindness and respect, just like you would treat your precious, innocent children.

That's right, your body is like an innocent child—it has no control over how you treat it.

You will protect your body just as you protect and care for those who depend on you to protect and care for them.

You can and you will be able to resist any craving for the unhealthy choices that have negatively affected your life and your well-being.

Your craving will grow steadily and markedly less, and it will rapidly reach an almost permanent zero level.

Your subconscious mind will begin to block much of the discomfort of craving the wrong kinds of food or too much food.

That's right, these messages will help you to cope with any desire to overeat. As your mind blocks your craving, your brain begins to change.

Your emphasis is upon your commitment to protect your health and it begins to feel natural to protect your body.

By protecting your body, you are gradually developing a temple of health through which you will experience your life.

That's right—you live each and every moment of your life through your body, and because you want that experience to be the very best possible, you will begin to respect and protect your body.

You will protect your body and begin to create a divine home for your spirit.

Each day, you will begin to experience greater pleasure through your body.

You will begin to appreciate what your body can do for you when you begin treating it with respect.

As you visualize your body being a source of pleasure and pride, just notice how good that makes you feel about yourself.

As you see yourself in a more slender form, notice how good you feel.

Be clear in your mind that this image that you hold of yourself at your ideal weight is completely realistic and attainable.

The more you believe in this image, the more natural the positive food choices become for you.

Spend several seconds now allowing that image to grow stronger and stronger in your mind's eye.

Notice how any image of an overeater simply dissipates from your mind.

That old, embarrassing image is fading away and is being replaced by a vibrantly healthy, more slender form in which you will begin to experience more pleasure and comfort.

You see yourself becoming more slender, more vibrantly healthy, and experiencing more pleasure through your body.

With that very pleasing image of yourself in your mind, take a deep breath and feel the confidence well up in your chest. With another deep breath, feel the psychological strength coursing through your veins.

Not because you are reading these words but because of the power of your subconscious mind you can and you will resist any desire to overeat.

No matter the circumstances, regardless of the situation you are going to maintain your new lifestyle changes and feel very good about yourself.

Chapter Ten

Lifestyle Change Suggestions

*"If we really want to live, we'd better start at once to try.
If we don't, it doesn't matter, but we'd better start to die."*
—W.H. Auden

As I said at the outset, this is not a diet book. However, I do want you to have specific strategies to make your lifestyle changes easier. Again, these are strategies I use personally. They have also worked well for many of my patients. Weight loss books geared toward honest, sensible weight loss have also provided helpful information. These lifestyle changes didn't happen overnight for me, and they won't for you either. But these suggestions will help you make the transition.

LIFESTYLE CHANGE COMMITMENT CONTRACT

One of the first things I ask my patients to do is sign a Lifestyle Change Commitment Contract. Get it in writing—it may add some incentive to stick with your lifestyle changes. The contract's wording also creates an attitude of acceptance to stick with the program in the face of inevitable difficulty.

Lifestyle Change Commitment Contract

I _____ agree to make every effort to maintain my lifestyle changes. I understand that my health and fitness are critical to my future well-being. I promise that, when I make mistakes, I will view them as learning experiences and *never* give up on my decision to change my lifestyle long term.

Signature _____ Date_____
Witness _____ Date_____

AVOID GUILT TRIPS

As you've promised if you signed the Lifestyle Change Commitment Contract, you will have inevitable slip-ups—which you will view as learning experiences. There are no real mistakes, only opportunities for learning.

This is a good place to use your cognitive restructuring skills. You can use positive self-talk statements to prevent further cheating. Statements like "I will not abandon my commitment to my lifestyle changes," "I will recover from this mistake,"

"Tomorrow will be a better day," and "I will remain strong in spite of my slip-up," are a great way to start.

The best way for me to handle slip-ups is to make up for them the next day. If I go a long time without a mistake, I actually give myself permission to cheat if I know I have earned it. A rare slip-up actually strengthens my resolve. The longer I have followed this program, though, the less frequently I even have the desire to cheat.

CHANGE THE FOOD YOU CONSUME

You will begin to lower your consumption of sugar, refined carbohydrates (i.e., white flour and white rice), and fried foods. You will learn to combine certain foods to get healthy, quality protein without consuming too much fatty meat. These changes may seem rather dramatic to you. But if you understand why consuming too much of these foods makes it so difficult to lose weight, you will be more motivated to lower your consumption.

LIMIT YOUR CONSUMPTION OF REFINED CARBOHYDRATES

There are several reasons why refined carbohydrates are among the foods I suggest you limit. Note that I said *limit*. It is virtually impossible to avoid these foods completely, but it will be to your advantage to minimize them.

First of all, the main reason white flour and rice are white is because the husks are removed, which also takes out most of the nutrients. The nutrients that are removed contain the fiber that we know is essential in aiding digestion. There is another reason that refined carbohydrates can be bad for you in terms of weight loss: by transforming the whole grain into finely ground flour, the surface area of the particles has increased greatly. Imagine the surface area of all those tiny flour particles versus that of one whole grain. It's a huge difference and causes the calories from bread made from white flour to be absorbed very quickly into your body—even faster than refined sugar— thus giving some bread a higher glycemic index than sugar. Also, the lack of fiber contributes to the immediate absorption into the body, making the glycemic index even higher and resulting in rapid secretion of insulin. This can exhaust the pancreas, potentially causing diabetes. There is also evidence that the food additives used in processing white flour adversely affect the body and alter moods.

The Wheat Food Council suggests one half cup of whole wheat flour and one half cup of all-purpose flour can be substituted for one cup of all-purpose flour in any recipe.

LIMIT YOUR CONSUMPTION OF REFINED SUGAR

No one needs to be told any more that refined sugar is bad for them, but a better understanding of why may increase your motivation to limit your consumption. When refined sugar was first introduced in Europe in the sixteenth century, it was rationed very strictly because of its believed potent, drug-like effect.

In 1975, William Duffy, author of *Sugar Blues*, stated that "refined sugar is lethal when ingested by humans." This may be a bit of an exaggeration, but you can see that the dangers of sugar have been known for quite some time. The authors of *Sugar Busters* suggest that "sugar just may be the number one culprit in lowering quality of life and causing premature death."

Sugar, like white flour, is absorbed immediately in a concentrated fashion, resulting in rapid insulin secretion, exhausting the pancreas—and, again, potentially leading to diabetes. In addition, too much sugar leads to exhaustion and depletes vital nutrient reserves, especially essential minerals and B vitamins. Sugar is found in a lot of junk foods and is high in calories, and, therefore, often replaces healthier foods in one's diet.

LIMIT YOUR CONSUMPTION OF FATTY RED MEAT

I also suggest that you limit your intake of fatty red meat. Although there is not much wrong with lean red meat, it contains very small amounts of trans fat, and there is no safe amount of trans fat that you can consume. Unfortunately, most meat consumed is not lean and would, therefore, contain more trans fat. The fact that mad cow disease is now in the United States is also worthy of consideration. It's another risk to think about as you choose your foods.

Also, I believe the typical western diet contains too much protein, and meat is the main culprit. It contains very little fiber, and high levels of protein can eventually lead to liver and kidney disorders.

There is also a great deal written about the whole process of feedlots—and growth hormones, antibiotics, and other chemicals given to the animals prior to their slaughter—and the effects of these on the people that eat the meat. This is worthy of consideration and concern. If you're going to eat red meat, buy it as lean as possible and as natural as possible. There are several good reasons here to get your protein primarily from other sources.

GETTING HIGH-QUALITY PROTEIN WITHOUT EATING MEAT

In order to get protein from non-meat sources, it is important to understand the makeup of protein. Protein is a molecule made up of a long chain of units called amino acids. Amino acids are known as the building blocks of protein.

There are twenty-two different amino acids, nine of which are essential. The essential amino acids cannot be synthesized in your body, but must be consumed in the food you eat. Non-essential amino acids are labeled as such because, if you do not get them from food, you can manufacture them yourself from fats, carbohydrates, and other amino acids.

Meat, eggs, and dairy foods are considered high-quality proteins, or *complete proteins*, because they contain a good mix of essential amino acids without any significant deficiencies. They are easily absorbed by the body and used to make new proteins efficiently. Even though animal foods have the right combination of amino acids, they have the various drawbacks discussed in the previous section.

Some plant sources of protein, however, as a single source do not contain all of the essential amino acids. But you can avoid the drawbacks of animal products and maximize the benefits of plant foods by combining certain foods—certain plant sources, to be specific—and eating them together. This is a process called complementarity—you basically combine a food that is deficient in one amino acid with a food that has plenty of the missing amino acid. You will make combinations such as legumes and dairy products, whole grains and legumes, whole grains and dairy products, and legumes and nuts or seeds. One of the best-known examples is rice and beans, the staple of many Mexican dishes.

One of my favorite recipes provides a good example of these combinations: lima bean pesto risotto. Instead of using rice, I use whole barley and get the same effect as using Arborio rice. Barley, the main ingredient, is loaded with the essential amino acid methionine, but has very little lysine. The lima beans have lots of lysine, but very little methionine. Adding a little parmesan cheese, which has an abundant amount of lysine and isoleucine, gives you another great combination.

The beauty of this kind of combining is that the value of the whole food is greater than the sum of the parts. This means that, by adding these various amino acids together, you actually increase the value of the individual amino acids.

INCREASE YOUR FIBER INTAKE

There is no question that increased fiber in your diet contributes to weight loss. Fiber reduces feelings of hunger, slows the pace of eating, reduces the caloric value of food (because part of it is fiber), and creates a feeling of fullness as you eat it.

Eating foods high in fiber makes you less likely to overeat because of the fullness they create in your stomach.

Fiber comes from plant foods, and there are two types: soluble and insoluble. Soluble fiber attracts water and can be found in nuts, seeds, barley, beans, oat bran, lentils, peas, and in some vegetables and fruits. Eating soluble fiber has been clinically proven to lower blood cholesterol and, as a result, lowers the risk for heart disease. Insoluble fiber can be found in whole grains, wheat bran, and vegetables. Some foods that are high in insoluble fiber are crackers and cereals made with whole grains, fresh fruits, and raw or slightly cooked vegetables.

Fiber slows the digestion of other foods, which has a positive effect on the glycemic index of those foods. It also off-sets some of the irritation of the body's digestion of fats in the intestines by helping to remove bile salts after digestion. This protects your intestines and the prostate from damage caused by the digestive juices.

Most naturally-occurring fat comes in foods that also contain natural fiber. Nature has done a marvelous job of creating foods that provide healthy fats that, at the same time, also provide high fiber content, such as nuts and seeds. It is important to realize that, when you eat foods that contain fat but contain no fiber, you also need to eat another high-fiber food along with the meal. Vegetable oils and fats from animal sources do not contain significant amounts of fiber, so these fats need to be complemented with fiber. It's not hard to do: for example, the fiber in a raw-vegetable salad is a healthy complement to the oil in the salad dressing. A salad with a chicken breast provides another good combination.

Something I have done for years that provides a healthy alternative to the typical white-flour pasta you buy at the grocery store is to look for whole-grain pastas such as rice, whole wheat, or quinoa. Some grocery stores carry it, but, more than likely, you will want to go to health food stores. I almost cannot tell the difference and, after doing it for so long, I actually prefer whole grain.

CONTROL YOUR ENVIRONMENT

By exercising some control on your environment—where you live, where you go, and with whom you spend your time—you will be able to minimize the difficult food choices you have to make.

Nola, a patient, said she doesn't feel like a good mother unless her freezer and cabinets are full of the foods her family members like. This includes food she knows is unhealthy. She is working toward limiting the amount of unhealthy food in her home, but it is very challenging for her. She is trying to see herself as a good mother for reasons other than indulging her family's wishes for unhealthy foods. Many mothers have also admitted to me that they tell themselves they are buying certain foods for their children but deep down know it is for their own consumption.

Debbie, a very social and outgoing person, says that she eats differently with different friends. At times, it seems that eating is the major source of entertainment for some of her friends. I have suggested that she may need to take a serious look at the friends she spends time with, especially the ones who actually encourage unhealthy eating.

When you go to the grocery store, be very mindful of what is going into your grocery cart. You can get a leg up on controlling what goes into your home by using discipline at the grocery store.

There is no question that buffets need to be eliminated from the environments you inhabit. If you absolutely cannot avoid them from time to time, don't fool yourself into thinking you have to get your money's worth. You are not saving money by eating yourself sick.

Also, if you eat at restaurants, you need to avoid fried and deep-fried foods as much as possible. Most restaurants use partially-hydrogenated vegetable oils in their deep-fat fryers, so those foods are loaded with trans fat. Margarines have trans fat and are often used instead of real butter. The portions in restaurants are usually bigger, so be aware of that.

GAIN SOCIAL SUPPORT

The literature is very clear on the benefits of social support. Among other things, social support has been shown to be an excellent buffer against stress, anxiety, and depression. Many people use social supports during difficult times. As E. S. Ford and others write, "Calling or talking to or being with someone is the best way of counteracting negative moods." As we've established, negative moods often cause people to overeat. If social support provides a buffer against those emotions, it could counteract your impulses to overeat.

When changing your lifestyle, you could experience various difficult emotions. Since food has been used at times as a numbing agent to these emotions, you may find it challenging to not go back to those old habits. Perhaps food has worked well for you from time to time to help you avoid difficult emotions.

If you have never gone the course or let yourself experience these emotions, how do you know what experiencing them might be like? Is it possible your coping skills are stronger than you realize? Your fear of these emotions may be disproportionate to the actual experience of them. As Mark Twain put it, "My life has been filled with many horrible things, most of which never happened." Doesn't reaching out to your social support seem to be a better alternative than eating? The difficult emotions will pass, as will the fear of facing them.

You will need to determine who your social support will be. They may be close friends, family members, or possibly therapists who sincerely want to support you in your endeavor to lose weight. These are people you seek out not only when you are feeling weak, but to whom you report your successes as well.

Just a quick telephone call to a friend can pick you up or possibly distract you from your craving or negative emotions. A hug, a pat on the back, or a word of reassurance from your spouse or family just might get you through a difficult moment.

For those of you who live with others, I suggest you explain to them what you are doing. Help them to understand that you plan to alter, within reason, the food that will be provided in the home. Ask for their understanding and patience. Some consideration on their part is reasonable to ask. In all likelihood, they will be willing to limit, to some extent, food no longer in your lifestyle.

DO NOT FORGET TO PUMP IRON

In the exercise section, I talked about the benefits of strength training, or weight lifting. I want to reiterate the necessity of balancing your aerobic training with some weight training. Professional opinions vary greatly on the amount considered adequate to contribute to weight loss. They recommend from as little as eight minutes a day to as much as one hour, three times a week. My recommendation is at least thirty minutes, three times a week. Make sure that when you lift the weight you are doing it at a steady, slow pace so as not to use any momentum that a faster pace might provide.

It is not necessary to join a gym in order to do strength training. There are medicine balls, elastic straps, appropriately sized hand weights, and many more methods for devising your own strength training at home. There are many books with instructions on how to get started. Many yoga poses provide methods for building muscle strength.

Weight training builds muscle, which speeds up your metabolism, thus burning calories. It improves your appearance by tightening the skin for a firmer look. Your skeletal system is supported by your muscles, so weight lifting improves your posture.

DO NOT WEIGH YOURSELF

In the year 2002, Americans spent $203.5 million on bathroom scales, up from $189.3 million in 2001. Wouldn't you expect that an increase in sales of an apparatus used to monitor and, ostensibly, control weight, might do just that? Unfortunately, just the opposite appears to be the case. As I have documented, the number of overweight individuals is steadily increasing, not decreasing. Here's my advice: stay off the scales!

I suggest that you use the clothing you are wearing to judge how you are doing. In my case, weighing only served to frustrate me. When I weighed myself, I was, of course, always hoping for good news. If my weight was down, I made the unfortunate mistake of rewarding myself by eating a little more than my lifestyle allowed. If, however, I had not lost any weight, I would often get discouraged and eat anyway.

Another reason I discourage weighing yourself too often is because many factors interact to affect the reading on your scale. Did you know that barometric pressure actually affects your weight? We normally weigh less in the morning; therefore the time of day will affect your reading. Women often retain a little water during the few days prior to and the first few days of their periods; therefore, the time of the month may change the numbers too. The food currently in your digestive system, as well as the clothing on your back, may also make a big difference.

If you are doing resistance training and aerobic exercise, you will begin to build muscle mass. Muscle, even though it takes up less body space, weighs more than fat. You can see how this might provide prime opportunity for discouragement, frustration, and, ultimately, falling off the wagon. Sometimes, your workouts cause your body to replace fat with muscle and to reproportion itself. You may not lose any weight on the scales when this happens, but you do lose fat, and you will find that your clothes fit better and you look better as a result.

For all of the above reasons, I consider the bathroom scale a rather evil contraption. In a matter of a few seconds, the numbers you see on your scale can change your feelings about yourself. Do not let your bathroom scale have that power over you. If you must weigh yourself, do it no more than once a week and always at the same time. Weigh yourself when you are completely nude.

DRINK WATER

Drink at least six eight-ounce glasses of water each day. Kirsch believes water to be so important that he calls it the "lost nutrient." Water speeds up metabolism, aids in digestion, and contributes to feelings of fullness. It also works to flush toxins from your system, which is especially good for a healthy-looking complexion. Water carries nutrients and energy to every cell in your body; it regulates body temperature, lubricates your joints, cushions your insides, and transmits electrical messages between cells. If all of that doesn't convince you to drink water, I don't know what will.

I recommend purified water, as do most nutrition experts. Unfiltered water contains chlorine, fluoride, and hydrocarbons, which may suppress thyroid function. Unfiltered water also requires the liver to work harder to filter and remove the additives.

EAT BREAKFAST

The majority of patients come to me as non–breakfast eaters. And, although I found no research to back it up, I believe that average to slim people are more likely to eat breakfast than overweight people. I did find a study showing that diet relapsers are more likely to skip breakfast. The reason it is so important to eat breakfast is to "break the fast," as the name implies. Because it has been several hours since you last ate, your blood sugar will keep dropping, and you are more likely to binge on whatever is available. It is also better to consume more food earlier in the day. Once you are in bed, your metabolism slows, and food eaten late in the day will drag through your system and be absorbed more fully.

LEARN TO DELAY GRATIFICATION

If you are going to lose weight, you are going to have to delay gratification from time to time. Be assured that every time you decline to eat something that is not part of your lifestyle, you will reap tremendous benefits not only from losing weight, but from feeling better about yourself. Also, remember that each decision you make to delay gratification strengthens those neural pathways that make delaying gratification easier the next time. In addition, when you do indulge after delaying gratification, the food will taste better, and you will be free of the guilt that only leads to further overeating. Remember, as you delay gratification to eat, you set up a healthy anticipation for your next meal.

SHARE AN ENTRÉE

When you eat out, you probably have a pretty good idea of the size of entrées the restaurant serves. There is nothing wrong with sharing a main course with your dining partner. I will often get my own salad and/or appetizer and then share an entrée. I don't believe I have ever come away from doing this and still felt hungry. It is also a good idea to ask for a doggie bag when you get full. Depending on the level of service, you may sit for a while before you get your check, and if a half-full plate is sitting in front of you, it may be difficult not to continue to nibble. I have asked for a doggie bag as soon as my entrée comes when I see that it is a large serving.

BE ASSERTIVE

Throughout this book, you've read about situations in which saying no to food offered by people in our lives was difficult. Learning to say no is probably the hallmark of assertiveness. The other part of assertiveness is asking for what you want.

Both learning to say no and asking for what you want are necessary ingredients to maintaining a healthy weight. Deficits in assertiveness are usually a result of putting others' feelings or needs ahead of your own. Remember, if you are overweight, you may get more pressure than your peers of normal weight.

SET A GOAL OF ONE POUND A WEEK

If you can lose one pound a week for one year, you will lose fifty-two pounds. That is a tremendous amount of weight. Many of you do not need to lose that much weight. You can see that, if you look for long-term weight loss and do not get hung up on losing a lot of weight right now, a year from now you can probably be at your ideal weight. Research is clear that slow, consistent weight loss is more likely to be permanent.

DO NOT BE FOOLED BY LOW FAT

In the early nineties, a very sad phenomenon occurred that wreaked havoc on millions of dieters in the United States. This was the low fat craze. Suddenly, everything came in low fat versions, and people were not only consuming more of these foods, but they were also beginning to eat reduced fat versions of foods such as potato chips and cookies from which they had previously abstained.

Another phenomenon was the idea of eating something low in calories as an excuse to eat other high fat foods. The idea that you can eat a double cheeseburger and French fries because you are drinking a Diet Coke with it is completely absurd. Despite its lack of calories, Diet Coke is no cure for the effects of trans fat on your body. Another example would be buying low fat salad dressing so that you can eat regular ice cream.

You must learn to read labels. Always look for trans fat, the partially hydrogenated oil that wreaks havoc on your whole body. Paradoxically enough, low fat and non-fat foods are often packed with sugar and calories. This sugar, if it is not metabolized, will turn to fat. Did you know that a regular serving of Oreos has 160 calories in a thirty-four gram serving, while a reduced fat serving of Oreos has 140 calories in thirty-three grams? As you can see, neither is something you want in your lifestyle very often. Again, always read the label to check for trans fat. Avoid that like the plague. When you see partially hydrogenated vegetable oil of any kind on the label, don't eat it. One or two grams (a thimbleful) of trans fat is worse for you than a whole cup of beef fat. Crackers, breads, pastries, and margarine are full of it. Don't eat them if it's in there. Even a trace amount is really bad for you. Eat real butter, not margarine or imitation butter spreads. Crackers are hard to find without trans fat. Even some of the so-called "fat free" brands like Keebler, when you read the label, will say they contain an insignificant amount. Nabisco fat free crackers, however, do not contain any trans fat.

LIMIT THE VARIETY OF FOODS YOU EAT

Even though I have included two weeks worth of meals in the following chapter, I do not think it is necessary to have that much variety in your regimen. Considerable research shows that those who maintain a healthy weight eat a more limited variety of foods. What is important is to find foods that you enjoy and stick to those. When you are trying to lose weight, it makes no sense to eat food you do not like just to increase your variety or because they are healthy. Save your calories for the foods you do like. Do your research, and find wholesome foods you like. When you eat food you really enjoy, you are more satisfied with less.

For example, I may eat salmon three times in a given week. I may have two or three tuna salad sandwiches in a week. I may also eat three arugula salads in one week. The point is to find healthy foods you like and do not feel as if you have to have a huge variety to get the nutrients you need.

Chapter Eleven

Menus and Recipes

"Behold, what I have seen to be good and to be fitting is to eat and drink and find enjoyment in all the toil with which one toils under the sun the few days of his life which God has given him."
—Ecclesiastes 5:18

Having read the first ten chapters of this book, you are armed with an arsenal of information to help you change your lifestyle. My hope is that what you have read has you excited and encouraged, and you are already incorporating it into your life.

I hope that you have given up the idea of finding yet another diet to follow and are truly motivated to make long-lasting lifestyle changes. You are probably much clearer about why you want to lose weight, as well as why you overeat. This information alone has the potential to radically change your approach to weight loss. You always knew that overeating was physically dangerous, but you now realize how much it is affecting you psychologically. You now know that you can do a great deal to control your mental attitude and health through better eating habits.

At the heart of this book is a radically new way of thinking about your ability to take the weight off once and for all. You are looking at your food urges and your ability to respond to them differently. You know that you can change your brain and actually get positive urges to work for you. I hope you are also seeing your body from a different perspective. I want you to see your body as something you cherish and from which you derive immense pleasure. With this new appreciation, you will find exercise to be more of a pleasure than a burden.

It is time now to look more closely at what you eat. In this chapter, I want to review carbohydrates, fats, and proteins briefly. I will give you some specifics about daily menus and several recipes. Even though I have included fourteen days of menus, the variety is much greater than you need. There is a lot of research that indicates that average-weight people do not eat an extensive variety of foods. My advice is that you find good, healthy meals that you like and stick with them. As I mentioned in the last chapter, I eat a tuna salad sandwich on whole grain bread with lettuce, tomatoes, and onions (no mayonnaise) two or three times a week. It is not unusual for me to eat salmon four times in a ten-day period. These are just a few examples, but I do not eat a huge variety of meals. It would probably take me three or four weeks to eat all of the meals included. Just pick the ones you really like and forget the rest.

When it comes to knowing what to eat, the U.S. Department of Agriculture's guide to good nutrition is probably the best available. The Food Guide Pyramid is based on years of research in human physiology. The authors of the guidelines admit that they are only recommendations and that there is room for individual considerations. They recommend that an American adult's dietary consumption consist of 55 to 65 percent carbohydrates, 20 to 30 percent fat, and 10 to 15 percent protein.

My recommendation is to be on the very low end of the total carbohydrate consumption, more in the 40 to 45 percent range. Increase your protein consumption so that your percentage is closer to the 35 to 40 percent range. I also recommend that you keep your percent of fat intake to around 20 percent.

Of course, not all carbohydrates, fats, and proteins are created equally. We will look at each individually, but certain guidelines apply across the board. To the extent that it is possible, foods that most closely resemble their natural state are superior. The fresher or more whole the food you consume, the better. Some examples of this are whole grain bread as opposed to white bread, lean steak as opposed to hamburger (unless it's 98 percent lean), fresh broccoli as opposed to frozen, real potatoes as opposed to potato chips, and fresh blueberries as opposed to blueberry preserves.

FOOD COMPONENTS
Carbohydrates

For the most part, the carbohydrates you want to consume are those that come from fresh fruits and vegetables and whole grains. You want to avoid carbohydrates that come from white sugar and white flour.

The glycemic index (GI) of various carbohydrates is a helpful concept to understand when choosing which carbohydrates to eat. This index refers to the speed at which the carbohydrate is converted to glucose and enters the bloodstream. High-glycemic foods are more likely to cause you to gain body fat by increasing the amount of insulin that is secreted, causing rapid absorption of glucose from the blood that gets stored as fat. Still, don't rely completely on GI when making choices. You still need to look at the calories. The following chart includes a glycemic index table for various carbohydrates.

Glycemic Index for Common Foods

HIGH	MEDIUM	LOW
Glucose 100	Apple Juice 41	Apple 36
Baked Potato 85	Banana (Ripe) 50	Barley 22
Corn Flakes 84	Banana Bread 47	Banana (Unripe) 30
Cheerios 74	Baked Beans 43	Black Beans 30
Corn Chex 83	Bran (All) 44	Brown Beans 38
Corn Flakes 83	Bran Chex 58	Butter Beans 31
Cream of Wheat 66	Brown Rice 59	Cherries 22
Dates, Dried 103	Corn 55	Chickpeas 36
Graham Crackers 74	Fruit Bread 47	Grapefruit 25
Grapenuts 67	Hominy 40	Green Beans 30
Grapenut Flakes 80	Ice Cream 50	Kidney Beans 27

Honey 73	Oatmeal 49	Lentils 29
Kaiser Roll 73	Orange 43	Milk (2%) 32
Puffed Rice 90	Orange Juice 57	Milk (Skim) 27
Puffed Wheat 74	Pinto Beans 42	Pear 36
Raisins 64	Pound Cake 54	Soybeans 18
Saltines 72	Popcorn 55	Soy Milk 31
Table Sugar 65	Pudding 43	Split Peas 32
Waffles 76	Special K 54	Spaghetti 40
Wheat Thins 67	Sweet Potato 54	Strawberries 32
White Bread 72	White Rice 56	Vermicelli 35
Whole Wheat Bread 72	Whole Wheat 41	Yogurt 38

Fats

Just as is true with carbohydrates, there are good and bad fats. Without question, fats are essential to good health. They perform important functions, including their role in building adipose (fatty) tissue. Adipose tissue, among other things, holds stored energy, helps to regulate body temperature, and cushions internal organs. Dietary fats also enable you to use fat-soluble vitamins (such as A), maintain cell membranes, enhance your sex drive, and much more. Fats also help to maintain the integrity of the skin, the structure of cell membranes, and synthesize certain hormones. Essential fat is also an important component of the brain, nerves, and retina, and its absence in the body can promote weight gain. Consuming the right type of fat can make a big difference in how the body loses weight and how well-equipped the body is to deal with weight loss.

Some fats are beneficial to health and promote weight loss, and some fats are a detriment to health and a barrier to weight loss.

By far the worst fat you can eat is trans fatty acid, or trans fat. It was first introduced into the home with Crisco in 1911. It is the only man-made fat in the food supply and experts agree that trans fat is a key factor of the obesity epidemic. Trans fat is made by partially hydrogenating vegetable oils in order to make them solid at room temperature for use in margarines and fake butter. This bombarding of relatively healthy polyunsaturated fat with hydrogen gas in the presence of a metal catalyst (nickel or platinum) creates fat molecules that are freaks of nature, so to speak. Natural fat molecules, which were once curved, get straightened out into a new shape. The shape of fatty acid molecules matters a lot because they stack together, and if you change the shape, you change how they stack and behave in the body. They are not easily broken down, and the body doesn't know exactly how to process them. They don't really fit into the natural cellular makeup. Researchers believe trans fat is one of the reasons cells malfunction. Trans fat may actually reprogram how cells work—how they talk to each other and function. Even just a few grams of trans fat a day is enough to gum up the workings of cells in the body. It has been shown to cause cancer and to interfere with the way insulin works in your body; it is also thought to lead to diabetes, high blood pressure, and high cholesterol, and it interferes with the way your body keeps the inside of your arteries and blood vessels clean. It can also cause beer belly, because that's where it goes if your body decides to store it.

Trans fat is abundant in grocery stores in processed foods, cereals, crackers, snacks, frozen potpies, and margarines—to name a few. Trans fat is also used in cookies, pastries, donuts, piecrusts, and other foods for the effect it has in certain recipes, and also because it is cheap.

Jeremy M. Felts, a chemist and weight trainer, offers a good description of fats and how they affect your body. Some of the chemistry terms may be a little over the head of the average reader, but it is clear and to the point, and well worth the read.

There are four primary types of fat, each with its own unique molecular structure: saturated, monounsaturated, polyunsaturated, and trans fats. Unlike protein and carbohydrates, which have around four calories per gram, each of these four types of fat has over nine calories per gram, and therefore should be used sparingly in the diet to help promote weight loss. However, fat should never be omitted from the diet completely.

Each of the four primary fats has a different effect on blood cholesterol levels, which has a great bearing on risk for heart disease. Cholesterol is measured as a ratio of LDL-to-HDL, as well as total cholesterol. In order to have the least amount of risk for heart disease, the ratio should strongly favor HDL over LDL. A person with high total cholesterol could therefore have a lower risk over another with a lower total score, but with a less favorable ratio. It is important to remember that that this ratio of "good" to "bad" cholesterol can be modified greatly by the intake of specific fats and the avoidance of others.

Saturated fat is a nonessential fat found mostly in meat and dairy products. It is a solid at room temperature. Saturated fat is called so because its carbon chain is saturated with hydrogen atoms and has no double bonds. Saturated fat raises total cholesterol by raising both HDL and LDL levels in the body. Due to its adverse effects relating to heart disease, this fat should be avoided or at least used sparingly whenever possible. It can be virtually eliminated from the diet if so desired, as it has no nutritional value, and competes for absorption with other fats.

Monounsaturated fat is a nonessential fat also known as omega-9 fatty acid. It is found primarily in olive oil, avocados, and nuts such as almonds, peanuts, cashews, and macadamia. Many recent studies have shown that a diet rich in monounsaturated fat raises HDL levels, thereby protecting the cardiovascular system from damaging atherosclerotic plaque caused in part by high cholesterol. Monounsaturated fat is burned as energy almost as easily as saturated fat, provided that there are adequate essential fatty acids present in the body. This healthy fat should be used as the primary fat in the diet, but still used sparingly, as it can promote weight gain just as any fat can in large amounts. A few tablespoons of cold-pressed extra virgin olive oil, half an avocado, or a handful of raw nuts per day should be enough to achieve the desired benefits of this heart-healthy fat.

Polyunsaturated fat is the type essential to the human body. Also called essential fatty acids, this type of fat cannot be replicated in the body; it must be consumed through food or supplement. Polyunsaturated fat lowers both LDL and HDL levels and works well in conjunction with monounsaturated fat. Polyunsaturated fat has two subtypes: omega-3 and omega-6.

As stated previously, these essential fats serve a variety of functions in the human body. One of the most important functions of essential fat is to serve as a building block for hormones. They are also found in brain tissue, nerves, retina, and cell membranes (which have the crucial function of transporting nutrients and waste in and out of the cells). Deficiency of essential fatty acids has been shown to make the body react as if it is in a state of famine. In this condition, it retains excess fat rather than burning it as energy.

Omega-3 fatty acids are the reason fish such as salmon has been touted recently as such a heart-healthy meal. Besides salmon, other sources of omega-3 fatty acids include fortified or free-range eggs, some wild game, and cold-water fish such as mackerel, herring, sardines, black cod, anchovies, lake trout, and albacore tuna. They are also found in flaxseed oil, walnuts, pumpkin seeds, hemp seed oil, and wheat germ.

Omega-6s are found in black currant seed oil, borage oil, and evening primrose oil, which can all be found at most health food stores. Healthy sources of other omega-6s include raw pine nuts, pistachios, sunflower seeds, and cold-pressed versions of soybean, sunflower, or safflower oil.

According to the FDA and countless other sources, there is no safe intake of trans fat; it should, therefore, be avoided at all cost. In addition to other adverse effects, trans fat lowers HDL while increasing LDL, which is the worst-case scenario in the fight against heart disease risk.

Trans fats are created by hydrogenating (or adding hydrogen atoms to) polyunsaturated vegetable oils, such as soybean or cottonseed oil, using heat and pressure. This process makes the oil more stable, giving it a longer shelf life and saving money, but it changes a manageable polyunsaturated fat into something the body is poorly equipped to handle, and much of the time does not know quite what to do with. The body attempts to utilize these faulty trans fats in the same manner as regular essential omega-3s and omega-6s, creating faulty membranes and hormones. It is no surprise that they have such profound detrimental effects on the body and its processes.

Trans fats can be found in a lot of the foods on grocery store shelves. It is also found in small amounts in red meat and dairy products, created as a byproduct of fermentation in the bovine stomach. Beginning in

January 2006 the FDA required special labeling on all packaged foods containing trans fats. It is imperative to read label ingredients to halt their purchase and consumption. The ingredients to be avoided will state "hydrogenated" or "partially-hydrogenated" vegetable oil or vegetable shortening. Being conscious about the amount and the type of fat consumed is important to weight loss, cardiovascular health, and cancer risk reduction. Consumption of fat can be an asset or detriment to overall health, depending on the choices made. An ideal diet would be to consume primarily monounsaturated fat and secondarily omega-3s and omega-6s in order to keep a favorable cholesterol profile and avoid essential fatty acid deficiency. Saturated fats can be consumed in very small amounts, but trans fats should be avoided at all costs. Read labels before food purchase and inquire about fat content at restaurants to make informed choices about the amount and type of fat consumed.

—Jeremy M. Felts, BA Chemistry, Weight Trainer

So do your very best to avoid trans fat at every opportunity. As mentioned earlier, even tiny amounts—a thimbleful—are harmful. You have to read labels to know if it's in the food, and if you see "partially hydrogenated" anything, don't buy it. Some food manufacturers are responding to the dangers, however, and are changing their products to be intentionally trans fat free. You can see it on the labels of some bread now. This is great. I hope that this will happen more and more, and one way to help it happen is for people simply to stop buying foods that contain it.

Primarily, you want to consume—sparingly—monounsaturated fat, which is found in olive oil, avocados, and nuts such as almonds, peanuts, cashews, and macadamia. And you can see that there are essential fatty acids. These are found in lots of different kinds of fish such as salmon, mackerel, herring, sardines, black cod, anchovies, and albacore tuna.

Protein

The adequate consumption of protein is extremely important. In fact, the word protein comes from the Greek word for "of first quality." Proteins make new cells, maintain body tissue, synthesize enzymes, synthesize neurotransmitters, synthesize hormones, and create DNA.

As you have learned, too much protein from animal sources is unhealthy. Good lean meat in small quantities is fine; however, there are probably better ways to get healthy protein than eating meat.

The breakfast menus that follow include several protein shakes. These shakes are an excellent source of protein, but I recommend that you drink them only on days you have exercised. It is also best to drink them as soon as you finish your exercise and not later in the day.

READY, SET, GO

It should be clear from reading this book that I think eating ought to be an enjoyable experience. The sample menus and recipes are not the low fat, low-calorie, no-taste meals that many assume are necessary for weight loss. The suggested menus and recipes may differ somewhat from the way you usually eat, but everything included is delicious and, at the same time, healthy.

You will notice that there is no white flour and very little refined sugar in my recipes. There are a number of meals that include brown rice. I try to cook a substantial portion of brown rice and freeze it. It takes whole grain brown rice about thirty minutes to cook, and it freezes well. If you have it on hand, you will not be tempted to use instant white rice as a substitute.

There are also no suggested snacks included in the menus. If you do snack, I recommend fruit, whole grain crackers (trans fat free), low fat yogurt, mozzarella cheese, and fresh, raw vegetables.

An additional disclaimer on the included menus and recipes has to do with the amount of food included each day. All of the meals are relatively healthy and low in fat and calories; however, I believe that if you ate all of the food over a two-week period it would probably be too much. It is necessary to intersperse very small meals into this food regimen—at least one day a week or a couple of meals a week. There are days when I know I am eating a big meal for dinner and I will eat very little for lunch. My lunch may consist of just eight to ten whole wheat crackers and a slice of mozzarella cheese. On days when I go out for a larger-than-normal lunch, I occasionally will just have a bowl of cereal for dinner.

Sample Menus

Day 1

Breakfast
Egg White Omelet (page 206)
½ grapefruit
6 oz. yogurt with ¼ cup fresh berries

Lunch
Vegetarian sandwich (open-face or half sandwich: 1 slice
    whole wheat bread, lettuce, tomatoes, avocado, bean
    sprouts, cucumber, and 1 slice reduced fat cheese)
1 cup Tomato Soup (page 220)

Dinner
Salmon fillet (coated lightly with olive oil and cracked
    pepper, charcoaled)
Mixed green salad with Classic Dressing (pg. 204)
Butternut squash

Day 2

Breakfast
½ cup Kellogg's Bran Buds
½ cup Kellogg's Bran Flakes
1 cup skim milk

Lunch
1½ cups Vegetarian Chili (page 214) served over ½ cup
  brown rice
Celery sticks

Dinner
6 oz. sushi-grade tuna steak
Steamed vegetables
Arugula Salad (page 206)

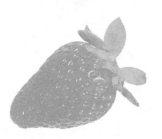
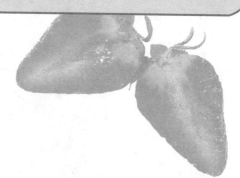

Day 3

Breakfast
Vegetable Frittata (page 207)
1 tangerine

Lunch
Thyme, Pea, and Egg Salad (page 208)
6 whole wheat crackers

Dinner
Vegetarian Lasagna (page 212)
Caesar salad

Day 4

Breakfast

Protein shake (Myoplex meal replacement powder in vanilla with ¼ cup strawberries, ¼ cup blueberries, 6 oz. orange juice, and 4 oz. water)

Lunch

Spinach Veggie Wrap (page 210)
1 cup mixed fruit (cantaloupe, honeydew melon, strawberries, and grapes)

Dinner

Marinated Shrimp and Mango Salad (page 209)
Asparagus spears

Day 5

Breakfast
2 poached eggs
1 piece dry whole wheat toast

Lunch
1 cup assorted red, yellow, and orange bell pepper slices
6 whole wheat crackers and 1½ ounces mozzarella
   cheese

Dinner
8 oz. halibut steak with Fruit Salsa (page 211)
4 tomato slices and 3 slices fresh buffalo mozzarella driz-
   zled with balsamic vinaigrette and garnished with lots
   of fresh basil seasoned with cracked pepper.
Steamed vegetables

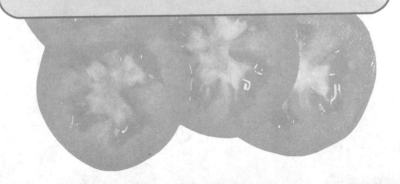

Day 6

Breakfast
Protein shake (see Day 4)

Lunch
Tuna-stuffed tomato
¼ cup raw almonds

Dinner
Salad with Raspberry Vinaigrette Dressing (page 204)
Lentil-Tomato Soup (page 211)

Day 7

Breakfast
Oatmeal

Lunch
Black Bean Salad (page 216)
8 whole wheat crackers
1½ oz. mozzarella cheese

Dinner
8 oz. grilled salmon
Vegetable Kebab (page 217)

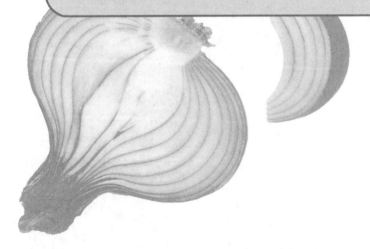

Day 8

Breakfast

½ cup plain old-fashioned oats (cooked in water)
¼ cup dried cranberries
¼ cup raisins
¼ cup skim milk

Lunch

Spinach salad with avocado and mango with Poppy Seed
  Dressing (page 205)
6 whole wheat crackers
1 oz. mozzarella cheese

Dinner

Shiitake Chicken Paillard (page 215)
Charcoaled Asparagus (page 209)
Caesar salad

Day 9

Breakfast
4 oz. grilled salmon
1 cup of mixed blueberries, strawberries, and raspberries
1 piece 100 percent whole wheat toast

Lunch
Red Beans and Rice (page 218)

Dinner
Fresh Tuna *Nicoise* Salad (page 219)
1 whole grain dinner roll

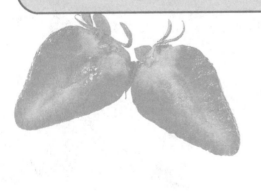

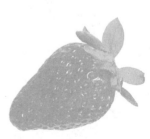

Day 10

Breakfast
Protein shake (see Day 4)

Lunch
1 cup Garden Vegetable Soup (page 221)
8 whole wheat crackers

Dinner
Shrimp and Scallop Kebabs (page 222)
Mixed greens with Classic Dressing (page 204)
(You may put the charcoaled fish atop the salad)

Day 11

Breakfast
1 cup Kashi GoLean Crunch cereal
¼ cup blueberries
½ cup skim milk

Lunch
½ cup Hummus (page 224)
1 cup assorted bell pepper strips
Raw almonds

Dinner
8 oz. salmon fillet (coated lightly with olive oil and fresh ground pepper, charcoaled)
Steamed mixed vegetables (broccoli, yellow squash, carrots, and snow peas)
½ baked potato, lightly buttered (When I eat a baked potato, I always discard about half of the meat of the potato and eat all of the skin.)

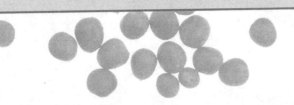

Day 12

Breakfast
2 poached eggs
1 piece dry whole wheat toast
½ grapefruit

Lunch
6-oz. chicken breast
Garden salad with Raspberry Vinaigrette Dressing (page
    204)

Dinner
Vegetarian Lasagna (page 212)
Caesar salad

Day 13

Breakfast
½ cup Kellogg's Bran Buds
½ cup Kellogg's Bran Flakes
½ cup skim milk

Lunch
Joyce's Gazpacho (page 224)
8 trans fat free crackers

Dinner
Sesame Shrimp and Vegetable Stir-Fry (page 220)

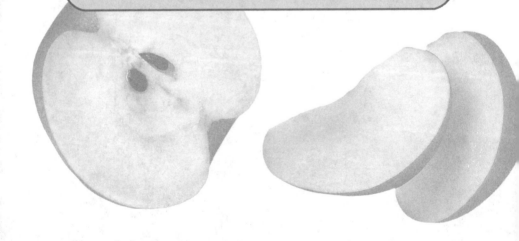

Day 14

Breakfast
Protein shake (see Day 4)

Lunch
Spinach salad with Raspberry Vinaigrette Dressing (page 204)
Garnish with rings of fresh red onion, sliced pear, and slivered almonds

---

Dinner
Kris Bryant's Southwestern White Chili (page 223)
Mixed greens salad with Classic Dressing (page 204)

Recipes

Classic Dressing

3 crushed garlic cloves
1 ½ tsp. Dijon mustard (or any sweet hot mustard)
5 tbsp. red wine vinegar
1 tsp. sugar
5 tbsp. olive oil
Fresh cracked pepper
Dash of salt

Combine garlic, mustard, vinegar, and sugar. Whisk briskly until sugar is dissolved. Slowly add olive oil and whisk gently until combined. Season with pepper and salt.

Raspberry Vinaigrette Dressing

Whisk together:
⅓ cup fresh orange juice
3 tbsp. raspberry vinegar
½ tsp. sugar
1 clove crushed garlic
Salt and freshly ground pepper to taste

Add ¼ cup olive oil and continue to whisk.

Poppy Seed Dressing

¼ cup white wine vinegar
3 tsp. granulated sugar
2 tsp. fresh lemon juice
¾ tsp. dry mustard
Salt to taste
⅔ cup trans fat-free vegetable oil (e.g., canola oil)
1 tbsp. poppy seeds

In a food processor combine the vinegar, sugar, lemon juice, dry mustard, and salt. Process on high. Add the vegetable oil and process on low. Remove from the processor and vigorously stir in the poppy seeds.

Balsamic Caesar Dressing

1 2-oz. can anchovy fillets, drained and coarsely chopped
3 tbsp. balsamic vinegar
1½ tbsp. low fat mayonnaise
1 tbsp. Worcestershire sauce
1½ tsp. minced garlic
Fresh cracked pepper to taste
¼ cup extra virgin olive oil
¼ cup grated pecorino Romano cheese

Put anchovies, vinegar, mayonnaise, Worcestershire sauce, garlic, and pepper into a food processor; process until finely chopped. With the machine on, add the olive oil in a steady stream. Add the cheese and pulse until just combined.

Arugula Salad

4 oz. arugula greens
Dress with 2 tbsp. olive oil and 1 tsp. lemon juice

Cut and peel one fresh pear, toss with greens and dressing.
Garnish with slivered parmigiano-reggiano cheese and drizzle with ½ tsp. truffle oil.

Egg White Omelet

3 egg whites
1 tbsp. skim milk
Fresh cracked pepper
1 tbsp. finely chopped green pepper, green onion, or any other fresh ingredients (e.g., fresh herbs like chives or basil)

Heat a small, nonstick skillet over medium-high heat and coat with olive oil cooking spray.

Whisk together the egg whites and skim milk. Season to taste with cracked pepper.

Add the egg mixture to the skillet and sprinkle with the fresh ingredients.

Cook for thirty seconds, or until edges begin to brown. Using spatula, loosen edges, fold omelet in half, and transfer to plate.

Vegetable Frittata

6 egg whites
3 whole eggs
12 oz. fresh asparagus spears
1 cup sliced fresh mushrooms
⅓ cup chopped tomato
¼ cup onion
¼ cup low fat cottage cheese
½ cup shredded cheddar cheese
2 tsp. prepared mustard
1½ tsp. snipped fresh thyme or tarragon
⅛ tsp. salt
Dash of pepper
Nonstick olive oil spray

Preheat oven to 400 degrees.

Steam asparagus until crisp and tender. Drain and reserve three spears for garnish. Cut remaining asparagus into one-inch pieces.

In mixing bowl, beat eggs until foamy. Beat in cottage cheese, mustard, thyme or tarragon, salt, and pepper. Stir in cheddar cheese and set aside.

Spray an unheated, large, ovenproof skillet with nonstick coating. Preheat over medium heat. Add onions and cook until translucent. Add mushrooms and cook until just tender. Stir in asparagus pieces. Pour egg mixture over vegetables.

Cook over low heat about five minutes or until mixture bubbles slightly and begins to set around the edges. Arrange fresh asparagus spears on top.

Bake uncovered in a 400-degree oven about ten minutes or until set. Sprinkle with tomatoes.

Makes four servings.

Thyme, Pea, and Egg Salad

⅔ cup frozen peas
1 hard-boiled egg
¼ cup chopped celery
2 tbsp. shredded, reduced fat cheddar cheese
1 tbsp. reduced fat mayonnaise
½ tsp. snipped thyme (⅛ tsp. dried)
Salt and pepper

In a mixing bowl, stir together the cheese, mayonnaise, and thyme. Add frozen peas, egg, and celery. Season to taste with salt and pepper. Cover and refrigerate for at least four hours.

Charcoaled Asparagus

Clean and trim asparagus

In large food storage bag, combine: 4 tbsp. balsamic vinaigrette, 1½ tbsp. olive oil, 2 crushed garlic cloves, 1 tsp. fresh thyme, 1 tsp. fresh rosemary, ½ tsp. fresh cracked pepper, salt to taste.

Add asparagus to bag and marinate for a few hours.

Charcoal over medium heat until tender. Brush asparagus with marinade.

Marinated Shrimp and Mango Salad

4 jumbo shrimp
Fresh garlic
Fresh ginger
Fresh parsley
½ orange juiced
½ lime, juiced
2 tbsp. red wine vinegar
Olive oil
Fresh cracked pepper
Peel and devein shrimp

In a small bowl, combine garlic, ginger, parsley, juice from orange and lime, vinegar, and olive oil. Coat shrimp with mixture, cover, and refrigerate for one hour to marinate. Grill shrimp over medium heat for two to three minutes per side.

Toss 4 oz. of mixed greens and a mango with Classic Salad Dressing (page 204).

Place charcoaled shrimp atop salad.

Spinach Veggie Wrap

1 eight-inch whole wheat tortilla (trans fat free if you can find it)
¼ cup avocado, smashed and spread on tortilla
½ cup fresh spinach
¼ cup fresh tomatoes
¼ cup mushrooms
⅛ cup chopped onion
1 slice Swiss cheese
¼ cup tomato salsa for dipping

Brown tortilla in a skillet on both sides. Top with avocado, spinach, tomatoes, mushrooms, onions, and cheese and place under broiler until cheese begins to melt. Roll tortilla up and cut in half. Serve with salsa for dipping.

Fruit Salsa

1 mango, peeled and diced
½ cup blueberries
½ cup strawberries, diced
½ cup red onion, finely chopped
3 tbsp. chopped fresh cilantro
3 tbsp. lime juice
2 tbsp. orange juice
3 tbsp. extra virgin olive oil
Salt and freshly ground black pepper

Combine fruit, onion, cilantro, juices, and olive oil. Season with salt and pepper. Let sit for thirty minutes at room temperature. May be refrigerated for one day. Serve at room temperature.

Lentil-Tomato Soup

1 cup dried lentils
5 cups water
1 onion
2 carrots, chopped
2 celery stalks, chopped with leaves
1 cup fresh spinach
1 cup fresh chopped tomato
Chopped parsley

Salt and pepper
Tarragon and thyme to taste
Dry white wine

Put first six ingredients into a large pot, simmering gently for about two-and-a-half to three hours, adding water if needed. Add ½ cup dry white wine. Add the fresh chopped tomato, parsley, and the spices to your liking and cook another twenty minutes.

Serves six.

Tuna Salad

1 can tuna
½ cup chopped celery
½ red onion
¼ cup sweet pickles, chopped
2 tbsp. low fat mayonnaise (trans fat free if you can find it)

Combine all ingredients and season with salt to taste.

Vegetarian Lasagna

For tomato sauce:
4 tbsp. olive oil

1½ cup chopped onion

2 tbsp. minced garlic

1½ cups chopped green pepper

4 tbsp. fresh basil (1 tbsp. if dried)

2 tbsp. fresh oregano (2 tsp. if dried)

3 bay leaves

2 tsp. salt

Sauté above ingredients; when onions are translucent, add:

2 13-oz. cans tomato puree

1 6-oz. can tomato paste

4 tbsp. dry red wine

1½ cups fresh chopped tomatoes

½ tsp. fresh cracked pepper

Cover and simmer for forty-five minutes.

Add: ½ cup fresh parsley

½ cup grated Parmesan cheese

1 cup fresh chopped spinach

Cheese mixture: 1½ cups ricotta cheese

1½ cups low fat cottage cheese

1½ tsp. salt

½ tsp. fresh cracked pepper

½ cup Parmesan cheese

1 lb. low fat, thinly sliced mozzarella

Layer:

Whole wheat lasagna noodles

Cheese mixture

Mozzarella cheese
Tomato sauce
Repeat layers.

Bake at 375 degrees for forty minutes. Garnish with mozzarella triangles. Let stand for ten to fifteen minutes before cutting.

Vegetarian Chili by Joyce

2 tbsp. olive oil
2 medium zucchini (cut into ½-inch cubes)
2 large red bell peppers, diced
2 onions, chopped
6 garlic cloves
2 jalapeño peppers, chopped
2 28-oz. cans chopped tomatoes with juice
1 15-oz. can Italian stewed tomatoes
2 tbsp. chili powder
1 tbsp. ground cumin
1 tbsp. dried basil
1 tbsp. dried oregano leaves
2 tsp. fresh cracked pepper
1 tsp. salt
1 tsp. fennel seeds
½ cup chopped parsley (fresh Italian if possible)
1 can dark kidney beans (drained and rinsed)

2 cans garbanzo beans
1 15-oz can hot chili beans
1 15-oz. can black beans
2 tbsp. dill weed
2 tbsp. lemon juice

Heat olive oil in soup pot and sauté onion, garlic, red and jalapeño peppers until wilted (ten minutes). Add zucchini and sauté five minutes. Add tomatoes, chili powder, cumin, basil, oregano, pepper, salt, fennel, and parsley. Cook uncovered, stirring often, for thirty to forty-five minutes.

Stir in all beans, dill, and lemon juice. Cook for another fifteen to twenty minutes and adjust seasoning to taste.

Garnish with sliced green onions and low fat cheddar cheese. May be served over cooked brown rice. Serves eight.

Shiitake Chicken Paillard

6 oz. boneless, skinless chicken breast
Salt and pepper
¾ cup (approx. 2 oz.) sliced shiitake mushrooms
1 clove garlic, minced
2 tbsp. balsamic vinegar
¼ cup chicken stock or low fat, low-sodium chicken broth
1 tsp. chopped fresh thyme

Place the chicken between sheets of plastic and pound with a meat mallet to ⅛-inch thickness. Season both sides of the chicken with the salt and pepper.

Heat a large, nonstick skillet over medium-high heat and coat with cooking spray. Place the chicken on one side of the heated pan. Place the mushrooms and garlic on other side. Cook chicken for two minutes or until browned. Turn and cook for three minutes or until the chicken is no longer pink. While the chicken is cooking, cook the mushrooms and garlic for three minutes or until lightly browned. Remove the chicken and mushroom mixture to a serving plate.

Add the balsamic vinegar, stock, and thyme to the pan. Bring to boil over high heat. Reduce the heat to medium-low and simmer for thirty seconds or until liquid slightly thickens. Pour over the chicken and serve immediately. Serves four to six.

Black Bean Salad

2 16 oz. cans black beans (drained and rinsed)
1 yellow bell pepper, diced
1 red bell pepper, diced
3 green onions, thinly sliced
2 plum tomatoes, seeded and diced
1 package (10 oz.) frozen shoe peg corn, thawed and drained
3 tbsp. extra virgin olive oil
4–5 tbsp. lemon juice

5 tbsp. minced fresh cilantro
1 tsp. black pepper
Salt to taste

Gently combine all ingredients.

Vegetable Kebab

Marinade:
    2 tbsp. olive oil
    3 tbsp. Balsamic vinaigrette
    1 large garlic clove, crushed
    ¼ tsp. cracked pepper dash
    Dash of salt
Marinate and place on four skewers:
    8 small broccoli florets
    8 artichoke hearts
    8 medium mushrooms
    1 large red onion cut into 8 pieces
    8 slices yellow squash
    8 cherry tomatoes

Charcoal until vegetables are just tender.

Red Beans and Rice

1 cup dried red beans

3 cups water

1½ cups chopped onion

3 garlic cloves chopped in large chunks

1 tsp. dried oregano

2 bay leaves

2 tbsp. chili powder

1 tsp. ground cumin

1 tsp. dried coriander

1½ to 2 tsp. crushed red pepper flakes depending on taste

½ cup tomato juice

1 cup cooked brown rice

Soak red beans overnight (at least eight hours) Drain beans and place in large pot. Add 3½ cups water. Bring to a boil over medium heat and cook for five minutes. Stir in next four ingredients, reduce heat, and simmer for one hour. Time may vary slightly; beans should be tender. Add chili powder, cumin, coriander, red pepper flakes, and tomato juice. Continue cooking for thirty minutes. Spoon over brown rice.

Serves six.

Fresh Tuna Nicoise Salad

Dressing:
  ¼ cup white wine vinegar
  ¼ tsp. wasabi powder
  1 tsp. fresh thyme leaves
  1 small shallot, trimmed and chopped
  2 tbsp. fresh ginger, chopped
  2 tsp. fresh basil, chopped
  ½ cup freshly squeezed orange juice

Combine all the above ingredients except the orange juice in a blender or food processor. Process until the shallot is finely chopped. Slowly drizzle in the orange juice.

6 cups mixed greens
8–12 asparagus spears
1 cup trimmed string beans
8 small new red potatoes thinly sliced
1 cup jicama, cut into strips
16 cherry tomatoes, halved
4 6-oz. Ahi tuna fillets, grilled rare

Coat greens lightly with dressing. Arrange on four large plates. Divide vegetables evenly among plates (place vegetables in bunches, e.g., all the potatoes together, leaving room in center for tuna). Place Ahi tuna fillet on top of greens inside the circle of vegetables. Serves four.

Tomato Soup

2 tbsp. olive oil
1 cup chopped onion
⅓ cup chopped celery tops including leaves
3 large garlic cloves, crushed
5 medium mushrooms, chopped
1½ lbs. canned diced tomatoes (puree 1 cup)
1 tsp. dried basil
½ tsp dried oregano
¼ cup fresh parsley
2 cups skim milk

Sauté onions, celery, garlic, and mushrooms in olive oil until tender. Add canned tomatoes, puréed tomatoes, basil, oregano, and parsley. Add skim milk and cook for forty-five minutes. Salt and pepper to taste. This is chunky and delicious and very healthy (Lots of fiber!).

Sesame Shrimp and Vegetable Stir-Fry

2 lbs. asparagus
3 tbsp. sesame seeds
2 tbsp. olive oil
1 medium onion
6 garlic cloves, chopped

1 medium red pepper
2 lbs. shrimp (shelled and deveined)
3 tbsp. low-sodium soy sauce

Steam trimmed asparagus and cut into two-inch pieces. Toast sesame seeds in skillet until golden and set aside. In same skillet over medium-high heat in hot oil, cook onion, garlic, red pepper, and asparagus. When vegetables are almost tender, add shrimp and cook until shrimp is pink, stirring frequently. Stir in soy sauce and then sesame seeds.

Serves four.

Garden Vegetable Soup

4 cups water
2 cups vegetable broth
1 cup chopped onion
1 cup chopped celery with leaves
¾ cup chopped green pepper
1½ cups shredded cabbage
1½ cups broccoli florets
1½ cups sliced small mushrooms
½ cup chopped carrots
¾ cup sliced zucchini
1 28-oz. can diced tomatoes
2 bay leaves

1 tsp. dried basil
1 tsp. dried oregano
½ tsp. dried lemon peel
½ tsp. salt
Fresh cracked pepper to taste

In large soup pot, combine all ingredients except zucchini. Bring to boil. Reduce heat, cover, and simmer for approximately one hour. Add zucchini after about forty minutes. Serve when all vegetables are tender. I always make plenty of this because if freezes well.

Serves eight.

Shrimp and Scallop Kebabs

12 scallops and 1 lb. of shrimp
Marinade:
   2½ tbsp. olive oil
   3 tbsp. dry Sherry
   1 tbsp. ginger freshly grated
   2 garlic cloves crushed
   ½ cup orange juice (freshly squeezed)
   Juice of two limes (freshly squeezed)
   1 tsp. salt
   Freshly ground pepper
   4 shallots, finely chopped

Wash and drain shrimp and scallops. Cover and marinate for one hour. Reserve marinade and brush fish while cooking. Cook until shrimp are pink.

Kris Bryant's Southwestern White Chili

1 tbsp. olive oil
1 lb. boneless, skinless chicken breast cut into cubes
¼ cup chopped onion
1 cup chicken broth
1 4-oz. can green chilies
1 19-oz. can white kidney beans, undrained
3 garlic cloves, crushed
1 tsp. ground cumin
½ tsp. oregano leaves
½ tsp. cilantro leaves
¼ tsp. ground red pepper

Heat oil in a two- to three-quart saucepan over medium heat. Add chicken and cook for four to five minutes, stirring constantly. Remove chicken with slotted spoon (cover and keep warm). Add chopped onion and garlic and cook for two minutes. Stir in the broth, green chilies, cumin, oregano, cilantro, and red pepper. Simmer for thirty minutes. Stir in cooked chicken and beans. Simmer ten minutes.

Hummus

1 16-oz. can garbanzo beans
¼ cup liquid from beans
3 garlic cloves, crushed
3 tbsp. lemon juice
2½ tbsp. tahini
1 tbsp. cumin
½ tbsp. cayenne pepper (season to your liking)

Combine in food processor and process to desired consistency. Garnish with extra virgin olive oil and paprika.

Joyce's Gazpacho

6 large ripe tomatoes, diced (vine ripened, if possible)
2 medium cucumbers, seeded and coarsely chopped
2 medium yellow onions, coarsely chopped
1 large shallot, coarsely chipped
2 red bell peppers
2 to 3 cloves garlic, crushed
1 large avocado, coarsely chopped
½ cup red wine vinegar
½ cup olive oil
1 cup tomato sauce
¼ cup packed minced parsley

1 tsp. salt
Lots of fresh ground pepper
1 tbsp. minced fresh basil

Combine tomatoes, pepper, cucumber, onion, and shallot in a large bowl along with garlic and parsley. Whisk together vinegar oil, salt, pepper, and tomato juice until well blended. Stir into vegetables with minced basil. Cover and chill for at least four hours. Serve chilled, garnished with avocado.

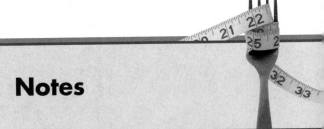

Notes

Chapter One. Hypnosis and Self-hypnosis for Weight Loss: Rewiring Your Brain

4 *"prolong a stay in consciousness"*: James, 429.

4 *"the mental faculty by which one deliberately"*: American Heritage Dictionary. New York: Houghton Mifflin Company, 2001, 931.

5 *"Cognitive-behavior therapy—"*: Schwartz, Jeffrey M., and Sharon Begley, 90.

Chapter Two. Learning to Think Differently about Losing Weight

29 *"Grief is the partner"*: Anderson, 85.

32 *"I need to keep discovering"*: Boorstein, 85.

33 *"not because I have"*: ibid, 86.

33 *Anticipated overeating actually leads to*: Ruderman, et al., 131-147.

39 *"becomes your own."*: Levine, 17.

Chapter Three. This is Not about Dieting

41 *"Dieting is a notoriously ineffective means"*: Heatherton, 118.

42 *"range from 75 percent to 95 percent"*: Consumer Reports. "Rating the Diets," Vol. 58(6), 354, June 1993.

45 *"food and drink regularly provided or consumed"*: Webster's Ninth New Collegiate Dictionary, 352.

49 *"based on a new nutritional principle"*: Polivy and Herman, 682.

49 *the success rate is actually higher*: Robinson, et al., 449.

49 *"feelings of frustration and defeat"*: Kassirer, et al., 53.

49 *big promises and repeat customers*: Polivy and Herman, 680.

50 *measurable improvement in distressed individuals*: Howard, et al., 161.

54 *Any diet book that claims permanent weight*: Bailey, 12.

55 *"choose a regimen that emphasizes"*: Fumento, 169.

Chapter Four. Why Do You Want to Lose Weight?

66 *"almost all women in the United States"*: Northrup, 607.

66 *"Society's standard of beauty is an image"*: Schneider, 67.

67 *41 percent of survey respondents*: Garner, 32.

Chapter Five. Why Do You Overeat?

85 *mild gurgling, gnawing*: Tribole and Resch, 72.

91 *obesity is often a result of emotional eating*: Ganley, 343.

91 *a special celebration gives us license*: Thayer, 57.

91 *"a constant often unconscious, inclination"*: Webster's Ninth New Collegiate Dictionary, 545.

Chapter Six. Overeating is Dangerous

101 *prejudice begins early in life*: Smith, 43.

Chapter Seven. Thinking about Your Behavior

115 *"Very recent research indicates that"*: Schwartz, 31.

118 *"appreciate that it is wonderful to be sitting here"*: Hanh, 159.

Chapter Eight. The Importance of Exercise

121 *"if you do just one thing, make it exercise"*: DeAnglis, 49.

131 *Working out first thing*: Shideler, 1D.

136 *"Technological society pushes us"*: Kornfield, 24.

138 *"a determination to submit your body"*: Smith, 149.

Chapter Nine. The Body as a Pleasure Source

144 *"You cannot do a single thing"*: Chopra, 168.

144 *"tool for living, the instrument"*: Yee, 7

149 *"at every stage of spiritual growth"*: Chopra, 167.

151 *"Our indefatigable pursuit of pleasure"*: Epsteub, 2.

Chapter Ten. Lifestyle Change Suggestions

160 *"refined sugar is lethal"*: Duffy, 47.

161 *"Sugar just may be the number one"*: Steward, et al., 47.

161 *Sugar, like white flour, is absorbed*: Ross, 35

166 *"Calling or talking to or being with someone"*: Ford, et al., 85.

169 *In the year 2002, Americans spent $203.5 million*: Garcia, D4.

Chapter Eleven. Menus and Recipes

183   *"There are four primary types of fat"*: Felts, "Fats and Other Suggestions Relating to Protein and Carbohydrates," Copyright 2003 Alexander & Fraser, Inc.

188   *"Proteins make new cells, maintain body"*: Rinzler, 100.

References

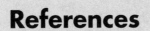

Anderson, J. *A Year by the Sea*. New York: Doubleday, 1999.

Boorstein, Sylvia. *Pay Attention, For Goodness Sake*. New York: Ballantine Publishing Group, 2002.

Callaway, Wayne. *The Callaway Diet*. New York: Bantam 1990.

Chopra, Deepak. *Ageless Body, Timeless Mind*. New York: Harmony Books, 1993.

Covert, Bailey. *The New Fit or Fat*. Boston: Houghton Mifflin, 1991.

Dass, Ram. *Still Here*. New York: Riverhead Books, 2000.

DeAnglis, Tori. "If you do just one thing make it exercise." *American Psychological Association Monitor* 33, No. 7 (2002): 49–51.

Duffy, William. *Sugar Blues*. New York: Warner Books, 1975.

Epstein, Mark. *Open to Desire: Embracing a Lust for Life*. New York: Gotham Books, 2005.

Ferguson, James M. *Habits Not Diets*. PaloAlto: Bell Publishing Company, 1988.

Ford, E.S., I.B. Ahluwaua, and D.A. Galuski. "Social Relationships and Cardiovascular Disease Risk Factors." *Preventive Medicine* 30 (2000): 83–92.

Fumento, Michael. *The Fat of the Land*. Yonkers, New York: Penguin Books, 1998.

Ganley, R.M. "Emotion and Eating in Obesity: A Review of the Literature." *International Journal of Eating Disorders* 8 (1989): 342–361.

Garcia, Leslie. "Pound Foolish." *The Charlotte Observer*, Mon, Apr. 07, 2003, D 4.

Garner, David. "Special Report: Body Image Survey Results," *Psychology Today*, February 1997: 30–34.

Germer, Christopher K. "Mantra, Intention and Psychotherapy." The Institute for Meditation and Psychotherapy. New England Education Institute Symposium, Santa Fe, NM. 2002.

Goodman, Trudy. "Introduction to Meditation." The Institute for Meditation and Psychotherapy. New England Educational Institute Symposium, Sanfa Fe, NM. 2002.

Hansen, Vikki, and Shawn Goodman. *The Seven Secrets of Slim People*. Carlsbad, California: Hay House Inc., 1997.

Heatherton, T.F., F. Mahamedi, M. Striepe, A.E. Field, and P. Keep. "A 10-year longitudinal study of body weight, dieting, and eating disorder symptoms." *Journal of Abnormal Psychology* 106 (1997) 117–125.

Howard, K.I., S.M. Kopta, M. Krause, and D.E. Orlinsky. "The dose-response relationship in psychotherapy." *American Psychologist* 42 (1986) 159–164.

James, William. *The Principles of Psychology*. Cambridge, Mass.: Harvard University Press, 1983.

Kassirer, J.P., and M. Angel. "Losing Weight—An Ill-fated New Year's Resolution." *New England Journal of Medicine* 338 (1998): 52–54.

Kirsch, David. *Sound Mind Sound Body*. United States: Rodale, 2000.

Kornfield, Jack. *A Path with Heart*. New York: Bantam Books, 1993.

Levine, Stephen. *Guided Meditations, Explorations and Healings*. New York: Anchor Books, 1991.

LeFever, Robert, and Marie Shafe. "Brain Chemistry: Combinations of Foods in the Blood Trigger Effects Very Similar to Alcohol." *Employee Assistance* 3, No. 8, March (1991).

Northrup, Christiane. *Women's Bodies, Women's Wisdom*. New York: Bantam Books, 2002.

Polivy, Janet, and Peter Herman. "If at First You Don't Succeed." *American Psychologist*, Volume 57 (9), September 2002: 677–689.

Rinzler, Carol. *Weight Loss Kit for Dummies*. New York: Hungry Minds, Inc.

Robinson, Jonathan I. et al. "Obesity, Weight Loss and Health." *Journal of American Diabetes Association* 93 (4) April (1993): 445-449.

Ross, Julia. *The Diet Cure*. New York: Viking Press, 1999.

Ruderman, A.J., L.J. Belzer, and A. Halpern. "Restraint, Anticipated Consumption, and Overeating." *Journal of Abnormal Psychology* 6 (1985): 131–147.

Sarwer, D.B., and T.A. Wadden. "The treatment on Obesity: What's New, What's Recommended." *Journal of Women's Health and Gender Based Medicine*, 8 (1999): 483–493.

Schneider, Karen. "Too Fat? Too Thin?" *People Magazine*, June 3 (1996): 64–74.

Schwartz, Jeffrey M., and Sharon Begley. *The Mind and the Brain: Neuroplasticity and the Power of Mental Force*. New York: Regan Books, 2002.

Schwartz, Jeffrey M., and Beverly Beyette. *Brain Lock: Free Yourself from Obsessive-Compulsive Behavior: A Four-Step Self-Treatment Method to Change Your Brain Chemistry*. New York: Harper Collins, 1997.

Schwartz, Jeffrey M., and Patrick Buckley with Annie Gottlieb. *Dear Patrick: Life is Tough—Here's Some Good Advice*. New York: Regan Books, 2003.

Scully, D., J. Kremer, M. Meade, R. Graham, and K. Dudgeon. "Physical Exercise and psychological wellbeing: A Critical Review." *British Journal of Sports Medicine* 32 (1998): 111–120.

Shideler, Karen. "How the Experts Keep Going." *The Wichita Eagle*, Oct. 29, 2002.

Sizer, Frances, and Eleanor Whitney. *Nutrition Concepts and Controversies*, 8th Edition. Stamford: Wadsworth/Thomson Learning, 2000.

Smith, Ian K. *The Take Control Diet, A Plan for Thinking People*. New York: Random House, 2001.

Steward, H. Leighton, and Morrison C. Bethea. *The New Sugar Busters: Cut Sugar to Trim Fat*. New York: Ballantine, 2002.

Thayer, Robert E. *Calm Energy: How People Regulate Mood with Food and Exercise*. New York: Oxford University Press, 2001.

Thich Nhat Hanh. *Anger*. New York: Riverhead Books, 2001.

Tribole, Evelyn, and Elyse Resch. *Intuitive Eating*. New York: St. Martin's Press, 1995.

Tzankhoff, S.P., and A.H. Norris. "Effects of Muscle Mass Decrease on Age Related BMR Changes." *Journal of Applied Physiology* 43 December 6 (1977): 1001–6.

"Varying the Intensity of Acute Exercise: Implications for Changes in Effect." *Journal of Sports Medicine and Physical Fitness* 35 (1995): 295–302.

Webster's Ninth New Collegiate Dictionary. Springfield Massachusetts: Merriam-Webster Inc., 1984.

Yee, Rodney. *Yoga, The Poetry of the Body*. New York: Thomas Dunne Books, 2002.

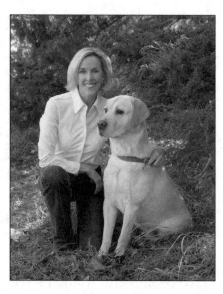

About the Author

Darcy D. Buehler, PhD, is a psychologist in private practice and has been helping people lose weight for more than eighteen years.

Dr. Buehler can be reached at her website drdarcybuehler.com. You can ask her questions and get feedback. Everyone can benefit from the support and individual attention the site provides. Since your feedback is invaluable, a questionnaire is on the site that Dr. Buehler uses to improve her methods.